M000282104

Cholesterol

The Real Truth

Are the drugs you take
making you sick?

Cholesterol: The Real Truth
Dr Sandra Cabot, & Margaret Jasinska ND

First published 2005 in Australia by WHAS
P. O. Box 689 Camden NSW 2570 Australia
02 4655 8855
www.whas.com.au

First published 2005 in USA by
SCB International Inc.
P O Box 5070
GLENDALE AZ 85312-5070
USA
Phone 623 334 3232
FREECALL 1888 75 LIVER

First Edition printed May 2005

Categories
1.Nutrition. 2. Diet 3. Cholesterol. 4. Heart Disease 5. Women's Health Advisory Service

Disclaimer
The suggestions, ideas and treatments described in this book must not replace the care and direct supervision of a trained health care professional. All problems and concerns regarding your health require medical supervision. If you have any pre-existing medical disorders, you must consult your own doctor before following the suggestions in this book. If you are taking any prescribed medications you should check with your own doctor before using the recommendations in this book.

Typeset by Christopher Martin
Illustrations by Christopher Martin

ISBN: 0-9673-9832-0

www.weightcontroldoctor.com
www.liverdoctor.com
www.whas.com.au

CONTENTS Contents

About the Authors

Dr Sandra Cabot MBBS, DRCOG,

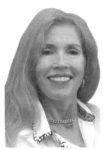

Sandra Cabot M.D. is a well-known medical doctor and author of the following best selling books:
• Hormones - Don't let them ruin your life. • The Body Shaping Diet • Hormone Replacement - the Real Truth (Balance your hormones naturally and swing from the chandeliers) • Boost your Energy • Raw Juices can save your Life • Can't lose weight? Unlock the Secrets That Keep You Fat • The Healthy Liver and Bowel Book • Liver Cleansing Diet.

Sandra is a consultant to the Australian Health Advisory Service, has regularly appeared in many national TV shows, and is developing her own Internet talkback radio show; writes for national health magazines and is a much sought after public speaker on nutritional medicine and hormonal disorders. Sandra is sometimes known as the "flying doctor" as she frequently flies herself to many of Australia's country towns to hold health forums for rural women. These help to raise funds for local women's health services and refuges. During the 1980s Sandra spent considerable time working in the Department of Obstetrics and Gynecology in a large missionary hospital in the Himalayan foothills of India.

With the publication of The Liver-Cleansing Diet in the United States of America, Sandra is at last able to share her significant experience and knowledge with men and women all over America.

Dr Sandra Cabot's books are available in America from bookstores and from SCB International Inc by calling 623-334-3232. Sandra has an office in Phoenix Arizona and you may phone her nutritionists on 623 334-3232 or visit www.weightcontroldoctor.com

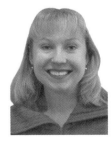

Margaret Jasinska ND, DBM

Margaret Jasinska is a naturopath who has been in clinical practice for seven years and now works very closely on a day to day basis with Dr Sandra Cabot. Margaret has a particular interest in disorders of the digestive and immune systems, as well as weight loss. She has researched the metabolic and nutritional influences on heart disease. Margaret is a keen writer, and enjoys keeping abreast of new developments in the health industry.

Margaret enjoys helping individuals improve their health through dietary modification and nutritional medicine.

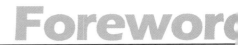

This book is controversial! It may ruffle some people's feathers and even provoke anger!

It is also impeccably well researched which enables us to base our recommendations upon a solid foundation of good nutritional science.

It takes courage to write a controversial book, which questions deeply entrenched conventional medical practices of the day. This book contains sometimes explosive information which is the opinions of the authors Dr Sandra Cabot and Margaret Jasinska ND, and in many instances your own doctor, drug companies and medical journals will not agree with its philosophies. In other words this book is not politically correct but we believe it is scientifically and ethically correct. The book has been written to make you think laterally and more deeply and this is good for your mind and body.

We believe that you will benefit by questioning your current treatment program in the following circumstances –

If you do not feel well despite being on cholesterol lowering drugs If you are experiencing side effects from cholesterol lowering drugs that are reducing your quality of life. If you are taking cholesterol drugs which are not working to control the symptoms or risk factors for a disease. If you have a deep down uneasy feeling about the long term consequences of the drugs you are taking. If you are taking drugs that you don't have enough information about regarding the way they work in your body. If you think that there may be an alternative equally effective, more natural and potentially safer way to control your risk factors for cardiovascular disease.

The fact that you have decided to read this book shows that you are not a passive accepting person, but rather an intelligent and aware person who likes to have some control over their health outcomes. So congratulations, as in this life your health is your greatest asset and you need to be vigilant and protective of this asset. I have found that many people who pay great attention to their financial assets and family members are often blissfully unaware of the side effects and risks of the things they put into their body – namely foods, chemicals and drugs. When I take a medical history I am often shocked that the patient has no idea about how the drugs they are taking work in their body and have never bothered to look up the potential side effects. I guess we tend to like a peaceful life and don't like to question professional people and upset the status quo. Also many of us are just too busy to do the enormous amount of research required to get ALL the facts, and indeed the infinite amount of information out there these days, especially on the Internet can be confusing, conflicting and is not always to be trusted. This is especially so if the information provider has a vested interest in you purchasing a product!

We the authors of this enlightening book have spent many years in clinical medicine and also doing academic research so that we can provide you with accurate and unbiased facts to give you a good understanding of the hot topic of cholesterol. We have done the hard work for you and tried to present the facts in a clear and enjoyable style. The topic of cholesterol is very complicated and over the past 20 years has been treated too simplistically and superficially. It is also a topic that is associated with the fear of heart attacks and strokes, and also billions of dollars in revenue; thus we can expect that people will have very definite and strong emotional viewpoints about it. We have not written this book with the aim of getting everyone to agree with our point of view but rather what we aim to achieve is that you will glean a greater understanding of the power of nutritional medicine.

If you have any questions you may phone Dr Cabot's Health Advisory Service on 623 334 3232 and speak to a health consultant. For contact details see www.weightcontroldoctor.com You will be very well informed after reading this book and this can only help you to communicate better with your own doctor and/or other health care provider. Of course you must stay under your own doctor's supervision and guidance because your doctor knows your history and intricate medical details. We are not encouraging you to stop any of your medications or change your current treatment program, as we do not know all your details. Some medications are much safer than others and indeed may be life saving. For example high blood pressure is a dangerous risk factor for heart attacks and strokes and medication is vital to control it. Generally speaking medications for high blood pressure are safe and well tolerated.

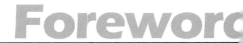

You must check with your own doctor before deciding to stop any medications, drugs or treatment and should let your doctor know what you are doing.

Introduction

Cholesterol: The Real Truth
Are the drugs you take making you sick?

Cholesterol is a topic that generates a great deal of interest, and also a great deal of controversy. Most of us become concerned about our cholesterol level as we reach middle age, and rightly so, since we are told high levels of cholesterol are a major risk factor for heart disease. Cardiovascular disease is the primary cause of death and disability in the United States. On average, one American dies of cardiovascular disease every 34 seconds. Ref. 1. 7,600,000 people have a heart attack each year in the US. That's an awful lot of people; I'm sure you don't want to be one of them.

If your cholesterol level happens to be elevated, your doctor will probably give you a stern look, advise you to improve your diet, (meaning eat less fat) and get some exercise. If that hasn't worked in a couple of months, you will probably be prescribed a cholesterol lowering drug.

Cholesterol is usually seen as the enemy; a harmful substance we must try hard to lower in order to halt the major killer of Americans: heart disease. This may not be the best advice, as cholesterol performs many vital functions in our body; in fact we could not live without it. There are also very real negative health consequences of lowering our cholesterol too far; these will be described in this book.

Isn't it strange that our grandparents' generation consumed far greater amounts of fat than most of us would dare to now? Butter, lard and dripping were often a common part of the diet. Why is it that now when we are all supposedly watching our fat intake, and opting for low fat varieties of foods, the incidence of heart disease is soaring?

There is much more to heart disease than just cholesterol. In fact, many researchers dispute the fact that high cholesterol has anything at all to do with heart attacks. Many of us know of somebody who was slim, appeared healthy, ate well, jogged each day and yet succumbed to a fatal heat attack fairly early in life. In fact 50 percent of victims of heart disease did not have any of the major known risk factors. Ref. 2. It doesn't seem fair! Perhaps there is much more to heart disease than we realize, and cholesterol is not the villain it is made out to be.

Recently scientists have discovered a whole host of measurable substances in our blood that are proving to be much stronger predictors of our risk of heart disease than cholesterol. Substances such as homocysteine, C-reactive protein, lipoprotein (a) and insulin all seem to be involved in the initiation and progression of heart disease, irrespective of our cholesterol level. In this book you will learn what each of these substances is, and how you can lower them if they are elevated. According to recent theories, inflammation seems to be the major trigger for the development of atherosclerosis (fatty plaques in the arteries). You will learn what causes inflammation, and what you can do to reduce it in your body.

Cholesterol lowering is big business. Drug companies make enormous profits on the sale of cholesterol lowering medications. Statins, (the most common category of cholesterol lowering drugs) are the biggest selling class of prescription medications. They earn their makers in excess of $US 20 billion each year. Ref. 3. Sales of the most popular statin, Lipitor reached $US 12 billion in 2004. Ref.4. Normal reference ranges for cholesterol levels have recently been lowered; this means that what was once considered a normal cholesterol level, is now considered too high. The result is that more and more people are being prescribed cholesterol lowering medication. This is coming at a huge cost to tax payers. In 2005, the estimated cost of CVD in the USA is $393.5 billion. Ref 5.

Because cholesterol has many vital functions in our body, it is not surprising that cholesterol lowering drugs have some nasty side effects. Most commonly they can cause muscle pain, liver dysfunction, memory and nervous system problems. Because cholesterol is needed for the manufacture of sex hormones, reducing your levels excessively may adversely affect your libido and sexual performance! Several studies have shown that certain cholesterol lowering drugs increase the incidence of cancer.

Why subject yourself to these side effects and make the drug companies rich, when there are plenty of safe, natural and effective alternatives to lower your cholesterol and reduce your risk of heart disease? This book will teach you how to take control of your health, and reduce the risk of becoming another heart disease statistic.

Chapter One

WHAT IS CHOLESTEROL AND WHY DO WE NEED IT?

What is cholesterol?

Cholesterol is a fat-like substance called a sterol. It is hard and waxy and melts at 300 degrees Fahrenheit . The name cholesterol originates from the Greek words *chole* (bile) and *stereos* (solid), as it was first discovered in solid form in gallstones. Our body manufactures approximately one gram of cholesterol per day; this is predominantly in the liver, but also occurs in the intestines, adrenal glands, ovaries and testes. In fact every cell of our body has the capacity to manufacture cholesterol if needed. We also obtain cholesterol in our diet by eating animal foods such as eggs, meat and dairy products.

Our body makes cholesterol out of a molecule called acetyl Co A; this is derived from the breakdown of sugars, fats and protein. Basically any calories in excess of our body's needs can be turned into cholesterol.

The following diagram details the manufacture of cholesterol.

Acetyl - CoA

▼

**3-hydroxy -3-methylglutaryl-CoA
(HMG-CoA)**

HMG-CoA reductase   ▼   **Statin drugs inhibit this step**

Mevalonate

▼

Isopentenyl-5-pyrophosphate

▼

Farnesyl-PP ◥

**heme a dolichol ubiquinone
(Co Enzyme Q 10)**

▼

Squalene

▼

2, 3 oxidosqualene

▼

Lanosterol

▼   **19 reactions**

CHOLESTEROL

◤   ◥

Bile salts   **Steroid hormones**

Cholesterol in Foods

Approximately 80 percent of the cholesterol in our body is manufactured in our liver. The remaining cholesterol is obtained through our diet. Only foods that come from animals contain cholesterol; plant foods such as vegetables, fruit, nuts, avocados and vegetable oil do not contain cholesterol. Plants do not have a liver, therefore it is impossible for them to contain cholesterol. The body makes much of its cholesterol out of saturated fatty acids in foods we eat. Saturated fat is found in foods like eggs, red meat and coconut, but it is also created in our body from the breakdown of sugar. Therefore, if we eat too much sugar, starch and carbohydrate rich foods, we will have a lot of saturated fat in our body, which can then be used to make cholesterol. Eating trans fatty acids raises our levels of bad cholesterol and lowers levels of good cholesterol. Trans fatty acids are present in most vegetable oil, unless it is cold pressed or extra virgin, as well as most margarines.

Below is a table with the cholesterol content of common foods:

FOOD	AMOUNT	CHOLESTEROL (mg)
Liver, chicken	3.5 oz	555
Egg	1	215
Prawns	3.5 oz	147
Crab	3.5 oz	127
Cheese, cheddar	3.5 oz	105
Lobster	3.5 oz	95
Salmon	3.5 oz	63
Pork	3.5 oz	62
Beef, lean	3.5 oz	60
Chicken, breast (skinless)	3.5 oz	58
Oysters	3.5 oz	47
Scallops	3.5 oz	45
Butter	1 tablespoon	35
Yoghurt, full fat	8 oz	32
Milk, full fat	8 oz	14
Margarine	1 tablespoon	0

| Egg white cooked | 1 | 0 |

Data adapted from Hepburn FN, Exler J, Weihrauch JL. Provisional tables on the content of omega-3 fatty acids and other fat components of selected foods. J Am Diet. Assoc 1986;86(6):788-792, and USDA Nutrient Data Laboratory.

Remember that just because a food is low in cholesterol doesn't mean that it is a healthy food; conversely many foods, such as eggs that are high in cholesterol are very good for us and can be included in the diet regularly. The cholesterol we eat has very little impact on our blood cholesterol levels.

Functions of Cholesterol

Cholesterol has many vital functions in our body, including:

- Membrane function. Cholesterol forms part of the cell membrane of each cell in our body. Because it is a hard fat, it gives the membranes rigidity and stability.

- Synthesis of steroid hormones. The sex hormones estrogen, progesterone, DHEA and testosterone are made out of cholesterol. This is a worry if millions of people are being prescribed cholesterol lowering drugs.

- Synthesis of adrenal hormones. The hormone aldosterone regulates water and sodium balance in our body and is made out of cholesterol. Cortisol is a hormone that regulates metabolism, suppresses inflammation and is produced as a response to stress. When we are under chronic stress our bodies manufacture a great deal more cholesterol.

- Bile production. 80 percent of the cholesterol in our body is used by the liver to produce bile salts. Bile is stored in the gallbladder and used to help in the digestion and absorption of dietary fats and fat soluble vitamins. This is the major route of exit of cholesterol from our body. Bile is secreted into our intestines and leaves the body in bowel movements.

- Vitamin D synthesis. Sunlight hitting our skin converts cholesterol into vitamin D, which is needed to keep our bones strong. Vitamin D has other important functions in our body; it boosts the immune system and helps to keep the blood pressure normal. Getting a bit of sunlight on your skin most days of the week can help to lower your cholesterol level by facilitating its conversion to vitamin D.

- Skin protection. Cholesterol is secreted into our skin, where it covers and protects us from dehydration, cracking and the drying effects of the elements. It helps to keep your skin looking plump and wrinkle free. Cholesterol has a role in healing, as high amounts of it are found in scar tissue.

- Serotonin function. Cholesterol is necessary for the function of serotonin receptors in the brain. Serotonin is a feel-good chemical that helps to protect us from depression. Several studies have shown that low cholesterol levels are associated with depression and violent behavior.

- Myelin sheath formation. Cholesterol is the main fat present in the myelin sheath, which coats our nerve cells and enables electrical impulses to occur in our brain and spinal cord. A healthy myelin sheath is needed for good concentration and memory.

- Antioxidant function. Cholesterol helps to transport fat soluble antioxidants around our body, such as vitamins E and A, and several antioxidant enzymes.

Cholesterol and other fats in Our Bloodstream

Cholesterol is not very soluble in water; therefore it must be carried around our bloodstream in various transport molecules. Certain proteins called apolipoproteins can wrap around cholesterol and other blood fats (lipids) to form what is called lipoproteins; these are essentially a combination of protein and fat. A description of the major fats in the bloodstream follows:

Chylomicrons
These are the largest lipoproteins, and mainly transport fat from the intestines to the liver. They mainly carry triglyceride fats and cholesterol which came from the diet, and those manufactured by the liver.

Very Low Density Lipoprotein (VLDL)
These are the lowest density lipoproteins because they are highest in fat; (the more dense the liproprotein, the more protein it contains). VLDLs are made in the liver and deliver triglycerides to various tissues, especially muscle (for energy production), and body fat (for storage).

Low Density Lipoprotein (LDL)
This is the so called "bad cholesterol". It is the major transporter of cholesterol and triglycerides, taking them from the liver to other parts of the body, where they can be used for various functions. You need your levels of LDL to be as low as possible.
There are other types of LDL:
Small dense LDL
This form of LDL is more likely to be taken up into the inner lining of arteries and promote atherosclerosis.
Oxidized LDL
This is what happens when free radicals cause damage to LDL molecules. This makes them more likely to promote damage to the inner lining of arteries, and for atherosclerosis to develop.

High Density Lipoprotein (HDL)

This is the so called "good cholesterol". It is high in protein, which makes it denser and lower in cholesterol. This lipoprotein takes cholesterol from various parts of the body to the liver, where it can be excreted in bile. HDL carries antioxidant enzymes and vitamins to prevent the oxidation of LDL cholesterol. You want your HDL to be as high as possible.

Triglycerides

These are a storage form of fat, made up of three fatty acids attached to a glycerol molecule. High triglyceride levels in the blood make it thick and sticky; they are a major risk factor for heart disease. Both excess carbohydrate and fat in our diet are converted into triglycerides in the liver.

Lipoprotein (a)

This particle is similar to LDL, but carries a sticky repair protein called apolipoprotein (a) which is used for tissue repair. It is a major risk factor for heart disease because it thickens the walls of the arteries.

Chapter Two

THE ROLE OF CHOLESTEROL IN HEART DISEASE

WHAT ROLE DOES CHOLESTEROL PLAY IN HEART DISEASE?

The idea that high cholesterol plays a role in the development of heart disease was started by the Framingham Heart Study. This study began in 1948 and monitored 5 000 healthy women and men living in Framingham, Massachusetts, USA. Researchers tried to establish which factors went on to determine if a person suffered a heart attack. High cholesterol was one factor that had some influence on who had a heart attack, but it was only one of 240 risk factors identified. Some other factors that influenced who got a heart attack included short stature, creased earlobes, male baldness, and being married to a highly educated woman!

Cholesterol was latched onto because it is a modifiable risk factor; that means there was an opportunity for drugs to be developed to lower cholesterol. There was potential to make great profits! Many scientists believe the results of the Framingham Study were misinterpreted, and cholesterol has been inappropriately focused on. The study only found an association between cholesterol and heart disease in young and middle-aged men; however over time we have all been instructed to fear cholesterol. Ref.6

In the late 1950s, researchers came up with the "lipid hypothesis", also known as the "diet-heart idea". This claimed there is a direct relationship between the amount of saturated fat and cholesterol in the diet, and the incidence of coronary heart disease. This hypothesis has received much publicity, and is the basis for why low fat, low cholesterol diets are the hallmark of nutrition recommendations. It is also the basis of prescribing cholesterol lowering medication to anyone who has levels above the desired limit.

Since then several researchers have discovered flaws in this hypothesis. Before 1920 heart disease was rare in the United States. This is a period of time when consumption of foods such as butter, lard and dripping was much greater than now; these are all foods very high in cholesterol. Many traditional diets of native populations are very high in fat and cholesterol, yet these populations have very low rates of heart disease.

The Masai tribes of Africa consume a diet of mostly milk, blood and beef; 60 percent of calories they eat are derived from fat. However, the Masai do not have elevated cholesterol, and are free of coronary heart disease. Inuit people (Eskimos) eat an extremely high fat diet; 80 percent of their calories come from fat. These people have healthy blood vessels and there is no evidence they suffered with heart disease. The traditional Australian aboriginal diet contained large amounts of fat in the form of eggs from birds and reptiles, turtles, eels and possums. Many insects are high in fat, such as witchety grubs (67% fat), the green tree ant and bogong moths; their abdomens contain a lot of fat. The aborigines were a fit and healthy population; obesity and diabetes were almost unheard of. Many researchers believe that it was the introduction of sugar, white flour and alcohol that has led to the explosion of diabetes, obesity and heart disease in this population.

One explanation for this contradiction is that the meat these native populations consumed was quite different in fat composition to the meat we buy from the supermarket or butcher today. Wild game meat is much lower in total fat, and particularly saturated fat than farmed meat. It is also higher in omega 3 essential fatty acids, which help your metabolism. This is why it may be a good idea to include game meat in your diet occasionally. Much of the fresh fish we purchase today is farmed, and unfortunately this type of fish is much lower in omega 3 fats than wild fish. This is because it is fed a type of "pet food", vastly different from the natural diet. Whenever you purchase fish, make sure you ask if it has been farmed or caught wild.

A very interesting study was published in the *American Journal of Clinical Nutrition*, highlighting the difference in rates of heart disease between people living in northern and southern India. The northerners ate a lot of meat, used ghee in their cooking and had high cholesterol levels. The southerners were predominantly vegetarians, they used vegetable oil and margarine to cook with, and they had lower cholesterol. You may be shocked to know that the vegetarians had a 15 times greater incidence of heart disease than the meat and ghee eaters! Ref.7. The explanation behind this is thought to be the replacement of traditional fats like ghee with modern, refined vegetable oils and margarine. Several years later, the *Lancet* reported that those living in northern India were developing more heart disease. Ref.8. The northerners had also been replacing ghee with supposedly heart healthy vegetable oil and margarine.

Proponents of the "lipid hypothesis" claim that when our intake of cholesterol and saturated fat is high, the saturated fat is turned into cholesterol which accumulates in the arteries. These deposits of cholesterol get thicker, form a plaque, and eventually narrow the arteries so much that blood flow is restricted. Plaques can also break off and form a blood clot in a vessel.

High levels of HDL "good" cholesterol protect us from heart disease by transporting excess cholesterol away from the arteries to the liver for removal. A high level of LDL "bad" cholesterol means that a lot of cholesterol must be depositing itself on the lining of our arteries, increasing our risk of heart attacks and strokes. This is true to a large extent, but is a very simplistic view of atherosclerosis (formation of fat plaques in the arteries). We now know there are many other factors involved.

Chapter Three

THE REASONS WHY YOU HAVE HIGH CHOLESTEROL

The most common reasons why your cholesterol is elevated

If your cholesterol level is elevated, these are the most likely explanations:

1. Poor Diet:

This is the most common reason why you may have elevated cholesterol levels. This is good news because it can be easily corrected. A high intake of fat and cholesterol in the diet is usually blamed for elevated blood cholesterol, but as you will learn, sugar and an excess intake of carbohydrate and trans fats are the real villains. Any excess calories we consume can be converted into cholesterol and triglycerides, therefore if you eat too much and become overweight, you raise your risk of heart disease. Changing what you eat is your most powerful weapon against heart disease.

a) Excess Carbohydrate
Today it is common for most people to eat a lot of carbohydrate. This is found in foods such as grains, cereals, starches and sugar. One reason for this is because we are constantly told to reduce our fat intake; we must eat something else to replace fat, and usually this means eating more carbohydrate. Another reason is because many people are addicted to carbohydrate. Sugar is addictive, and the more we eat it the more we crave it. Carbohydrate rich foods are also quick and convenient. A common diet may consist of toast or cereal for breakfast, a sandwich for lunch, pasta, rice or potatoes for dinner, and cookies, crackers or other sweets as snacks – not forgetting sugar in tea or coffee throughout the day.

It is true that we need carbohydrate for energy, but most of us are not athletes, and our sedentary lives never allow us to burn off this carbohydrate. Instead it is converted into body fat. It is also true that we are better off consuming complex carbohydrates, meaning it is better to eat wholegrain bread and pasta, and brown rice instead of their white, refined alternatives. However, this still usually results in too much carbohydrate in the diet, which is broken down into glucose.

When we get an excess of glucose into our bloodstream our body converts it into fat. Therefore, a high carbohydrate intake stimulates the production of fatty acids, which are joined together to form triglycerides. A high alcohol intake also raises cholesterol and triglyceride levels. You will learn that triglycerides are a major risk factor for heart disease. We all know that saturated fats are a really bad type of fat for our hearts. In fact not all saturated fats are bad; you can read about different types of saturated fats in chapter 4. It is the long chain saturated fatty acids that are bad for our heart because they are sticky, and can therefore clog our arteries. You do not have to eat any fat at all to have high blood levels of these saturated fats because our body makes them out of excess sugar in our diet. These fats can then be converted into cholesterol. So now you know that eating too much sugar, starches and grains can raise your levels of cholesterol and triglycerides, putting you at great risk of heart disease. If you do not burn off this extra fat through physical activity, you will not only appear overweight; fat deposits will accumulate in organs such as your liver, pancreas, heart, kidneys and other organs. Fatty degeneration of organs can occur as a result of excess sugar intake. Fatty liver disease now affects approximately 20% of the population. You can read how to overcome fatty liver in the book called *"The Liver Cleansing Diet"*.

b) Trans Fatty Acids

Some fats are good for our heart, some fats are bad, and some are terrible. Trans fatty acids are the worst kind of fat you could eat. You may have heard of these fats, as they have been receiving a lot of publicity lately. They are believed to greatly increase the risk of heart disease and cancer. We will go into more detail about the structure of fats in chapter 4. For now just briefly, unsaturated fatty acids in their natural state have a *cis* configuration. This means that at the position of the double bonds between carbon atoms in the fatty acid molecule, *both hydrogen atoms attached to the carbons are on the same side of the molecule.*
In trans fatty acids, *the hydrogen atoms attached to the carbons are on opposite sides of the molecule.* The word trans means across, or on the other side.

The diagram below illustrates this:

Cis- *Configuration*
Bent Molecule

Trans- *Configuration*
Straight Molecule

The twisting of the unsaturated fatty acid molecule to create a trans fat occurs when the oil is heated to high temperatures, such as during frying and deep frying, and also during the commercial manufacture of vegetable oil and some margarines.

Hydrogenation

The process of hydrogenation converts a liquid vegetable oil into a more solid state. This occurs through forcing hydrogen atoms into a vegetable oil under high pressure and high temperatures (248 to 410 degrees Fahrenheit). A metal catalyst is used; it may be nickel, copper or platinum, and the process takes six to eight hours. Hydrogenation may be complete or partial.

Complete hydrogenation is where this process continues until all the double bonds in the oil are saturated with hydrogen. In effect this creates a fully saturated fat which is now very hard at room temperature. Because there are no more double bonds, there are no trans fatty acids in this type of fat. This means that the fat is not as harmful to health as partially hydrogenated oil; however all essential fatty acids in the oil have been destroyed. Commonly tropical fats such as coconut fat and palm oil undergo this process, to make them more useful to food manufacturers. This is the type of vegetable fat that is often used in chocolate to make sure it melts at mouth temperature.

Partial hydrogenation is where the process is halted before the oil is totally saturated. This means the resulting fat is not as hard; it has a semi solid, spreadable texture. Many trans fatty acids are present in partially hydrogenated vegetable oil. The essential fatty acids in the oil are also damaged. The word "partially hydrogenated vegetable oil" is present on the label of very many processed foods. This type of fat is present in most margarines, vegetable shortening and processed food such as cakes, cookies, donuts, crisps and fries.

Are there any benefits of hydrogenated oils?

These types of fats benefit the food industry greatly, but our health suffers as a consequence. Usually cheap oils are used for this purpose, such as canola, cottonseed, soy or corn oil, which generally do not have health benefits. It is usually too expensive to use olive oil in manufacturing processed food. Hydrogenated fats, being solid give some foods the required consistency; cookies for instance are usually made from a solid fat like butter or margarine. Butter is more expensive to use than margarine, and it spoils much faster. Basically hydrogenated vegetable oil is used by the food industry because it is cheap, and gives the foods containing it a longer shelf life.

McDonalds replaced beef tallow with partially hydrogenated soybean oil in 1990. In September 2002 McDonalds promised to use healthier oil in its US stores by February 2003. However, nothing has been done so far; there are still six grams of trans fat in a large serve of fries. Ref.9. French fries are cooked in partially hydrogenated soybean, corn, canola, cottonseed, and/or sunflower oil.

The problem with vegetable oil

The vegetable oil you buy in the supermarket to cook with has usually been through a number of processes that have damaged the beneficial fats once present in the oils, and produced some toxic substances. Most oils come from seeds, nuts or fruit. Polyunsaturated and monounsaturated vegetable oils are quite delicate and unstable. This means that they are easily damaged and go rancid quickly. This can make them quite harmful to our health. Currently most vegetable oils are extracted in factories through the use of heat and chemical solvents. They are exposed to light and oxygen during processing, which negatively affect the oil.

The manufacture of cooking oil involves the following processes:

- The addition of NaOH (sodium hydroxide) to remove the alkali-soluble minor ingredients from the oil. The minor ingredients have health benefits, but diminish the shelf life of the oil; therefore they are discarded. Incidentally, NaOH is a corrosive chemical used to burn clogged sinks and drain pipes open.

- H_3PO_4 (phosphoric acid) is added to remove the acid-soluble minor ingredients. These also have health benefits, yet would lead to faster spoilage if left inside. H3PO4 is a corrosive acid used commercially to degrease windows.

- Bleaching clays are used to obtain greater shelf stability. The clays damage the molecules that give oil its color. Color absorbs light, and the light would lead to a faster deterioration of the oil. Bleaching makes the oil rancid, which gives it a bad odor and flavor.

- Consequently, the oil is then deodorized. This takes place at frying temperatures (428 to 473 degrees Fahrenheit). The resultant oil is colorless, odorless and tasteless.

Here are some of the minor ingredients removed from the oil during manufacture because it is not profitable to leave them in:

- Antioxidants including vitamin E and carotenes.

- Lecithin; which emulsifies oil and makes it easier to digest.

- Phytosterols; which you then pay high prices for in cholesterol lowering margarine.

- Chlorophyll; which has a blood purifying effect, and is high in magnesium.

If you cook with these kinds of processed vegetable oils and heat them to high temperatures, you are further destroying them and adding to the quantity of trans fatty acids they already contain. These kinds of processed vegetable oils are widely found in foods you may eat such as salad dressings, cookies, crisps, and crackers; basically wherever you see the words "vegetable oil" on the label. Extra virgin olive oil is not extracted or processed in this way. The health giving properties of the oil remain intact; therefore, if you must cook with oil, you are best off using it.

The problem with margarine

Margarine is made from the kind of processed vegetable oil described above, plus the oil is usually partially hydrogenated, like in the process described above. You will find that recently margarine tubs contain quite a few health claims; some margarine contains added omega 3 fats, some contain added vitamins or plant sterols, and some contain olive oil. It doesn't matter what kind of oil the margarine was made from; it is the oils used to make them, and the process of turning a liquid oil into something that is harder and spreadable that makes margarine an unhealthy food. Just about all margarines claim to be free of cholesterol. This is misleading because margarine is made out of vegetable oil, and no vegetables, nuts or seeds contain cholesterol anyway. The problem with margarine is the trans fats it usually contains which have the ability to raise cholesterol levels. You can read more about margarine in chapter 11.

Detrimental effects on health of vegetable oil and trans fats

Polyunsaturated fatty acids are more unstable than monounsaturated and saturated fatty acids. This means that they become rancid (oxidized) more easily when exposed to oxygen, light and heat, and have the ability to form trans fatty acids. We are continually told by health authorities that polyunsaturated fats are healthy, and saturated fats are bad for us.

Vegetable oils that have become oxidized act as free radicals in the body. Free radicals can cause damage to our cells and DNA; they age us more quickly and have been linked to the development of heart disease and cancer. Importantly, new research has shown that cholesterol itself is not the problem, but oxidized cholesterol is a bigger risk factor for heart disease. The more free radicals we have in our body, the greater the chance that our cholesterol will become oxidized. This form of cholesterol behaves differently and is more likely to attach itself to our artery walls.

Trans fats have been well researched in recent years, and their effects on our heart are becoming clearer. Some researchers believe they are responsible for the epidemic of heart disease in the 20th Century. Ref.10. Trans fats have an adverse effect on our blood fats because they increase the levels of LDL "bad" cholesterol, and reduce levels of HDL "good" cholesterol. This is a double whammy; their effects on cholesterol levels are considered to be twice as bad as saturated fats. Ref.11 This is very unfortunate because many consumers buy foods that are labeled to be "low fat" or "cholesterol free", and these are the types of foods that are often highest in trans fats! Trans fats are also known to raise triglyceride levels, and interfere with the metabolism of essential fatty acids in the body. Ref.12

In the Nurse's Health Study, women who had the greatest amount of trans fats in their diet had a 50% higher risk of heart attack compared to women who consumed the least amount of trans fats. Ref.13

Because trans fats become incorporated into our cell membranes, they interfere with the action of insulin. They promote insulin resistance and in this way they make you fat, and increase your chances of developing Syndrome X and diabetes. Trans fats also promote the release of inflammatory chemicals called cytokines, contributing to inflammation in the body.

If you do nothing else for your heart, make sure you avoid eating partially hydrogenated vegetable oil, and processed vegetable oil that does not state it is "extra virgin" or "cold pressed". In the USA the trans fat content of all packaged foods will need to be stated on the label by January 2006. Check food labels carefully to make sure you avoid these types of fats. Healthier alternatives to use would be extra virgin olive oil, butter, ghee and virgin coconut fat. Healthy spreads for bread include avocado, hummus, tahini (sesame seed paste), tomato paste or natural nut butter/paste.

The Donut Dilemma

The perfect donut requires that partially hydrogenated vegetable oil be used for deep frying. The United States FDA has stated that there is no safe level of trans fats in the diet, and ordered all food companies to disclose the trans fat content of their foods by January 2006. Many consumers are very aware of the dangers of trans fats, and actively avoid foods containing them. This has sent donut makers in America on a frantic race to come up with an alternative cooking oil for this popular treat.

Bob Pitts, of America's Dunkin' Donuts has spent the last year experimenting with 19 alternative cooking oils in his test kitchen near Boston. Things are not looking good; so far the donuts have turned out too heavy, or they just didn't taste good, or the donuts were so slick that the icing slid straight off them! Ref.14 Many US food processors have already spent tens of millions of dollars trying to get rid of trans fats from their junk food, without altering the taste of the product too much. The pressure is expected to intensify leading up to January 2006 when the labeling law comes in.

Finding an alternative to partially hydrogenated vegetable oil has turned out to be much more expensive than food companies first imagined. The oil is smooth, making it ideal for cream filled biscuits, and when used by fast food restaurants for deep frying, the oil can withstand repeated heatings, which saves money. Some food manufacturers have reverted back to using palm oil. This is high in saturated fat and was taken out of many foods in the 1980's because of an effective campaign to turn Americans off tropical fats for fear that they cause heart disease. This campaign was assisted by the American Soybean Association. Now we know that saturated fats are not as bad as the trans fats that replaced them. Who knows what food manufacturers will come up with to replace hydrogenated vegetable oil; let's hope it won't be something that turns out to be even more harmful.

c) Lack of Fiber

The main way our body gets rid of excess cholesterol is through our bowel movements. The liver pumps excess cholesterol that is not needed into the bile, which is stored in the gallbladder. Bile then enters our intestines through an opening called Vater's ampulla and leaves our body in bowel movements. If there is not much fiber in our diet, we don't drink enough water and are constipated, cholesterol in bile can get reabsorbed back into our bloodstream and we end up with high cholesterol levels. Therefore, one of the best ways to lower your cholesterol is to ensure that you have regular bowel movements.

The best kind of fiber for lowering cholesterol is soluble fiber. This kind of fiber becomes a gel-like consistency in the intestines, and it is able to bind with cholesterol and other toxins in our intestines and carry them out of our body. Good sources of soluble fiber include oats, legumes such as kidney beans or chickpeas, rice, barley, apples, strawberries and citrus fruits.

Another benefit of fiber is that it slows the absorption of sugar into our bloodstream when we eat some in our meal. This means that fiber lowers the glycemic index of a meal. This is good for reducing your risk of Syndrome X or diabetes, both major risk factors for heart disease.

2. Syndrome X:

Also known as metabolic syndrome, this condition is gaining greater awareness. 40-50 percent of men and women over the age of 50 have Syndrome X. Mexican Americans have the highest age-adjusted prevalence of Syndrome X. You can usually spot someone with Syndrome X by their round tummy. It is a metabolic disorder whereby 3 or more of the following conditions are present in the one person:

- Abdominal obesity, or excess fat in and around the abdomen. This means a waist circumference of >40 inches in men and >35 inches in women.

- Blood fat disorders (dyslipidemia). This is usually high triglycerides (≥150mg/dL) and low HDL cholesterol (<50mg/dL in women & <40mg/dL in men).

- High blood pressure (130/85 mmHg or higher)

- Insulin resistance or poor glucose tolerance. This usually means an elevated fasting blood sugar level of ≥110mg/dL.

- Prothrombotic state (ie. Tendency to form blood clots). This usually involves high fibrinogen or plasminogen activator inhibitor 1 in the blood. Ref.15

Syndrome X is usually caused by a diet high in carbohydrate, genetic factors, being overweight, certain medications and not doing enough exercise. As well as increasing your risk of developing heart disease, many people with Syndrome X go on to develop Type II diabetes.

How does Syndrome X put us at increased risk of heart disease?

When we eat carbohydrates (grains, starches, sugar), our body digests these into glucose (blood sugar). Glucose is a source of energy, and our body must decide how much of it to burn straight away, and how much to store for later use (as glycogen). The hormone insulin is released soon after we eat a carbohydrate containing meal, and its job is to help the glucose enter our cells, where it can be used for energy.

Once our glycogen stores are full, insulin converts the excess glucose we have consumed into fat, called triglyceride. High triglyceride levels are a major risk factor for heart disease, and triglycerides are deposited as body fat. Therefore, the hormone insulin can make us gain weight.

The type of diet we have greatly affects our blood insulin levels; diets high in sugar and foods made of white flour promote more insulin compared to diets consisting of vegetables and protein. Eating a lot of carbohydrate will release a lot of glucose into the bloodstream. Our body compensates for this by releasing a flood of insulin.

What Happens In People With Syndrome X?

Over time, their insulin becomes less and less effective. Insulin levels have been so high for so long, that the cells of the body (particularly muscle and fat cells) start to ignore it. It's like if someone continually talks and talks and talks; eventually you stop listening! So we can say the cells of the body have become resistant to insulin.

Initially, after a rise in blood glucose levels, the cells do not respond to the insulin that is released. The body responds by pumping out more and more insulin. Some hours later, when the insulin finally does work, there is a too rapid drop in blood sugar levels. This can make you suffer with hypoglycemia.

These are some common symptoms of hypoglycemia:

- Fatigue and feeling sleepy
- Mental fogginess
- Depression or anxiety
- Strong cravings for carbohydrates or sugar
- Hunger, even soon after a meal
- Feeling shaky or dizzy
- Sleep disturbances

All of these symptoms can make you want to reach for more carbohydrate, and hence the vicious cycle continues. This is why carbohydrates and sugar are often described as addictive! The desire to eat more carbohydrate can be overwhelming. It is usually the comfort foods people reach for to self medicate themselves when experiencing the symptoms of hypoglycemia, especially depression.

If Syndrome X is left to progress, you are at greatly increased risk of developing type 2 diabetes. As insulin becomes less and less effective, it has poorer control of our blood sugar; thus the blood sugar level becomes elevated. Diabetics have a much higher rate of heart disease than the general population.

Syndrome X and diabetes are the biggest risk factors for heart disease. You may remember from chapter one that the enzyme in the liver that manufactures cholesterol is called HMG-CoA reductase. This is the enzyme that cholesterol lowering drugs called statins inhibit. Interestingly enough the hormone insulin stimulates the activity of HMG-CoA reductase, causing it to manufacture more cholesterol. So now you see that the more sugar and carbohydrate you eat, the more insulin you secrete, and the more cholesterol your liver manufactures. Rather than taking cholesterol lowering drugs with potential side effects, wouldn't it just be easier to lower the amount of carbohydrate you have in your diet? You can have a blood test to measure your levels of insulin. You can read about this test in chapter ten. If you feel that you do have Syndrome X, you can read more about this condition, and follow an eating plan specifically designed to treat it in the book called *"Can't Lose Weight? Unlock The Secrets That Keep You Fat"*. For more information on Syndrome X please call our Health Advisory on 623 334 3232.

3. Genetic factors:

Often heart disease runs in the family, and sometimes large numbers of family members die at a relatively young age of this condition. Our genes affect how high our LDL cholesterol is because they determine how fast LDL is made and removed from the blood. You are two to five times more likely to have a heart attack if a first degree relative has died of coronary heart disease before the age of 60. Ref.16

There is a genetic condition called familial hypercholesterolemia (FH). It is an autosomal dominant disorder that produces severe elevations in total and LDL cholesterol. The DNA in our cells is packed into chromosomes, which occur in pairs. Autosomal comes from the word "autosome" which means all chromosomes other than the sex chromosomes. Dominant means that only one parent needs to contain the defective gene to pass it on to their offspring.

Heterozygous familial hypercholesterolemia occurs in approximately 1 in 500 people worldwide, and it causes an approximate doubling in LDL cholesterol levels. Ref.17 Heterozygous means that only one defective gene is present for a condition, so it usually produces a less severe case of the disease. In other words only one parent passed the condition on, rather than both parents. FH is especially common in French Canadians, Lebanese, South Africans and Ashkenazi Jews.

In FH the LDL receptors are either missing or deformed. These receptors are required in order for the liver to take up LDL that has been floating in the bloodstream, process it and remove it from the bloodstream. If the liver can't take up LDL particles, blood levels quickly rise. Also, if LDL is not able to get into liver cells, it can't suppress the production of more cholesterol, therefore greater amounts of cholesterol are produced, and blood levels rise. In people with heterozygous FH, only half the normal number of LDL receptors are present. Commonly, levels of LDL cholesterol will be between 199 and 402mg/dL. In normal healthy people LDL cholesterol should be no higher than 130mg/dL. People with heterozygous FH typically develop premature coronary artery disease; men typically in their forties, and women 10 to 15 years later.

Homozygous familial hypercholesterolemia is a much more severe case of the disease, as both genes are defective. It affects approximately one in one million people. In people with this condition sudden death due to a heart attack occurs as early as age 1 to 2 years.

High blood levels of LDL cholesterol in people with FH means that various cells in the body that do not require LDL receptors, take up and absorb cholesterol. This includes monocytes and macrophages, which can turn into foam cells and lead to the production of fatty plaques in the arteries.

People with familial hypercholesterolemia often display telltale signs on their bodies called xanthomas. The word xanthoma is derived from the Greek word *xanthos*, which means yellow. Most xanthomas have a yellowish appearance, but this isn't always the case. They are basically

deposits of fat, connective tissue and blood vessels in and under the skin which grow on various sites of the body. People with familial hypercholesterolemia typically develop xanthomas on their Achilles tendons and tendons on the hands. Sometimes a xanthoma develops on the inner side of the eyelid; this is called a xanthelasma.
An iridologist looking in the iris of a person with FH will usually see an arcus senilis, this is a cloudy ring on the outer border of the iris.
There are several other genetic conditions besides FH which produce severely elevated levels of LDL cholesterol.

4. Hypothyroidism:

This is a condition whereby the thyroid gland is under active. When the thyroid cannot produce enough T4 and T3 hormones, metabolism slows down; consequently the ability to process cholesterol is also impaired. Studies have shown that subclinical, or hidden hypothyroidism may be responsible for elevated cholesterol levels. Ref.18 Ref.19

Possible symptoms of hypothyroidism include:
- Weight gain
- Fatigue
- Depression
- Dry skin
- Hair loss
- Constipation
- Sensitivity to cold
- Muscle cramps, joint pain

If you suspect that you have an under active thyroid gland, ask your doctor for a blood test checking your levels of Thyroid Stimulating Hormone (TSH). This is a hormone produced by the pituitary gland in the brain, and if elevated, your thyroid gland may not be able to produce enough hormones.

5. Stress:

Studies have shown that chronic stress raises the risk of heart disease. One possible reason is that psychological and physical stress lead to the release of adrenaline; this causes the release of inflammatory cytokines such as IL6 and IL10. These are a kind of immune system chemical released by white blood cells which promote inflammation in the body, and can promote the development of atherosclerosis. Ref.20 Ref.21 The hormone cortisol is also released in response to stress. Chronically elevated levels of cortisol are related to high cholesterol, high triglycerides, high blood pressure, abdominal obesity and glucose intolerance. Glucose intolerance is a major risk factor for diabetes, and diabetics have higher rates of heart disease. Cortisol is a steroid hormone made out of cholesterol, therefore the more stressed we get, the more cholesterol gets made in our body.

When people feel stressed, they often adopt unhealthy habits. Overeating, binging on sweets, smoking and drinking more alcohol are common ways people deal with stress; each of these factors can raise our cholesterol levels.

6. Lack of exercise:

Leading a sedentary lifestyle is a major risk factor for several diseases, including obesity, heart disease, stroke and diabetes. Vigorous exercise that makes you huff and puff and break out into a sweat is one of the best ways to raise your levels of HDL "good" cholesterol and lower LDL "bad" cholesterol. Ref.22 Studies have shown that exercising for approximately 30 minutes, between three and five times a week elevates HDL cholesterol levels.

Regular physical activity helps to keep you lean, and improves blood sugar control, thereby reducing your risk of developing Syndrome X and diabetes. Aerobic exercise also strengthens your heart and makes it more efficient. If we exercise regularly, our coronary arteries expand more and are wider than the arteries in people who do no exercise. This means our heart gets a better blood supply and we are less likely to suffer with a heart attack.

7. Smoking:

Smoking is a well known major risk factor for heart disease, and several other diseases. It is capable of raising LDL cholesterol Ref.23 as well as blood pressure levels. Nicotine stimulates the release of the stress hormone adrenaline, which in turn stimulates lipolysis (fat breakdown) and increases blood levels of free fatty acids. These then stimulate the liver to release VLDL and triglyceride into the bloodstream. Smoking may lower levels of the protective HDL cholesterol, and chemicals in cigarettes cause damage to the artery walls, making it more likely for fat deposits to accumulate there.

Smokers have a 70 percent greater chance of dying from coronary heart disease than non-smokers. Smoking doubles the risk of having a stroke, and women who take oral contraceptives and smoke have a ten times greater risk of having a heart attack. Ref.24 However, there is hope because according to the World Health Organization, the risk of having a heart attack, stroke or peripheral artery disease drops significantly after the first two years of quitting.

Chapter Four

TYPES OF FATS AND THEIR ROLE IN HEALTH AND DISEASE

An Education in Fats

Many people are confused about fat; most of us are aware that there are bad fats and good fats, however advertising can give us the wrong ideas about which types of fats are healthy. Fat provides us with a concentrated source of energy, as it is very high in calories. Fat forms our cell membranes and acts as building blocks for hormones and other substances in our body. Fat is also needed to carry fat soluble vitamins in our body, including vitamins E, A, D and K. Basically, fats, (also known as lipids) are composed of fatty acids. There are several different types of fats we can obtain in our diet, and that are found in our body.

What is a fatty acid?

Fatty acids are chains of carbon atoms with hydrogen atoms filling up available bonds. Most of the fats in our body are triglycerides, which are three fatty acids attached to one glycerol molecule. Fatty acids can be classified as saturated, monounsaturated and polyunsaturated. This is determined by the presence of double bonds between carbon atoms.

Saturated fatty acids contain carbon atoms that are joined together by single bonds. There are no double bonds between carbon atoms, and each remaining position on the carbon atoms is taken up by a hydrogen atom, so we can say the molecule is saturated with hydrogen atoms. Saturated fatty acid chains can be between four and 28 carbon atoms long. These fatty acids are highly stable, meaning they do not readily react with other molecules, and they do not easily go rancid, or go off. They tolerate heat well, and do not oxidize easily. Saturated fats are usually solid at room temperature. They are commonly found in animal foods such as butter, suet, tallow, and tropical fats like coconut and palm oil. Our body makes saturated fats out of sugar and carbohydrate we have ingested. Saturated fats are the ones most blamed for raising cholesterol and causing heart disease.

The diagram below is of the saturated fatty acid butyric acid. It is common in butter. Notice how there are no double bonds between the carbon atoms in the chain.

Monounsaturated fatty acids have one double bond between carbon atoms in the carbon chain. This means that two hydrogen atoms are missing. They are usually liquid at room temperature and become solid when refrigerated. Monounsaturated fats are also fairly stable, and do not go rancid or oxidize easily; this means they can be used in cooking. The most common monounsaturated fat in our diet is oleic acid. It is found in large quantities in olive oil and consists of a chain of 18 carbon atoms; there is a double bond between carbons 9 and 10. Oleic acid melts at 55 degrees Fahrenheit , which is why in the fridge, or on a very cold winter's day olive oil can appear cloudy and solidified. Other oils high in monounsaturated fats are peanut oil and canola oil. You can see the structure of oleic acid below.

Polyunsaturated fatty acids contain two or more double bonds between carbon atoms in the chain. These fatty acids are liquid at room temperature, and even when refrigerated. They have a very low melting point. The most common polyunsaturated fats in our diet are linoleic acid, which has two double bonds and is also called Omega 6, and alpha-linolenic acid, which has three double bonds and is also called Omega 3. Omega refers to the position of the first double bond, so for example, in linoleic acid the first double bond starts at carbon 6. Omega 6 fats are abundant in popular vegetable oils such as sunflower, safflower, sesame and corn oil. These are promoted as "heart healthy" oils. Omega 6 fats are also found in evening primrose oil, and Omega 3 fats are found in flaxseed oil and fish oil.

The diagram below is of the Omega 6 fat linoleic acid; notice the two double bonds between carbon atoms in the chain.

The problem with polyunsaturated fats

Double bonds contain unpaired electrons, and polyunsaturated fats contain the most double bonds. This means they make the oil highly unstable whereby it can easily become rancid or oxidized. Polyunsaturated fats easily react with oxygen, light, water and various molecules in the body. If they become oxidized, such as through heating and exposure to oxygen (such as in processing and frying), polyunsaturated fats act as free radicals in the body. They can cause a great deal of harm in our bodies by damaging cell membranes and DNA. Damage to DNA may promote the development of cancer; free radical damage to our skin promotes wrinkles, and damage to blood vessels can promote the development of atherosclerosis. For this reason, polyunsaturated fats should never be used for cooking; yet these are precisely the oils sold in the supermarket specifically labeled for cooking!

All fats and oils in nature contain a combination of saturated, monounsaturated and polyunsaturated fatty acids. Animal fats like butter, cream and tallow contain mainly saturated fatty acids and plant fats contain mainly monounsaturated fatty acids, or polyunsaturated fatty acids. In their natural state, that is, when found in raw nuts and seeds, polyunsaturated fats are very healthy. However, when turned into vegetable oil via processing, polyunsaturated fats can do more harm than good.

Various health authorities claim that the typical Western diet is too high in omega 6 fats (present in most vegetable oils) and too low in omega 3 fats (present in fish, flaxseeds and walnuts). This imbalance may promote inflammation, contribute to weight gain, suppress the immune system and promote depression.

Length of fatty acid chains

Fatty acids can be classified based on their length, and this gives them different properties.

Short-chain fatty acids contain between four and six carbon atoms and are always saturated. Examples include butyric acid, containing four carbon atoms and present in butter, and capric acid, containing 6 carbon atoms and found in goat milk. Short-chain fatty acids have an anti-microbial effect in our digestive tract; they help to protect us from infections by bacteria, viruses and yeasts. They do not need bile to get digested; they are absorbed straight through our intestines and can be used straight away for energy.

Medium-chain fatty acids contain between eight and 12 carbon atoms. They are commonly found in butterfat and tropical oils like coconut fat. These fats also do not need bile to be digested, thus provide a quick source of energy. You may have heard of medium chain triglycerides (MCTs) used in the diets of people with digestive or liver diseases. They are also sometimes used by athletes, and are popular because they require very little digestive effort, and are quickly burnt off as energy, not stored as fat. They also have antimicrobial properties. Coconut fat is very high in **lauric acid,** which is a medium-chain fatty acid. In our body lauric acid is turned into monolaurin; this fat has antiviral, antibacterial and antiprotozoal properties. It acts to destroy lipid coated viruses such as herpes, influenza, cytomegalovirus, HIV, some bacteria such as listeria and Helicobacter pylori, as well as protozoa including giardia lamblia. Unrefined, or virgin coconut fat is an excellent addition to a healthy diet.

Long-chain fatty acids contain between 14 and 18 carbon atoms, and they may be saturated, monounsaturated or polyunsaturated. One example of an 18 carbon saturated fatty acid is stearic acid; it is found mainly in beef and lamb fat. Long chain saturated fatty acids are solid at body temperature and are sticky. If we consume large amounts of this type of fat, our bloodstream can become sticky, placing us at greater risk of heart disease. Our body can actually convert refined carbohydrates and sugar we have eaten into long chain saturated fatty acids. Therefore, eating a lot of sugar increases the amount of saturated fat and cholesterol in our body.

An example of an 18 carbon monounsaturated fatty acid is oleic acid, found in olive oil. The Omega 6 essential fatty acid linoleic acid, and

the Omega 3 essential fatty acid alpha-linolenic acid are both long chain polyunsaturated fatty acids, with 18 carbon atoms each.
Very-long-chain fatty acids contain between 20 and 24 carbon atoms. These include the Omega 3 essential fatty acids found in fish; eicosapentaenoic acid (EPA) and docosahexaenoic acid (DHA), as well as arachidonic acid (AA), found mainly in red meat. Most of these fats are used in the production of prostaglandins; hormone like substances in the body.

Plant sterols and stanols are also called phytosterols, and have a very similar structure to cholesterol. Plant sterols are found in the oils of plants such as nuts and seeds. The major plant sterol is called beta-sitosterol. Sterols are often refined and concentrated and added to margarines which claim to lower cholesterol levels. They can help to lower our cholesterol level by competing with cholesterol for absorption in our intestines. You can read more about cholesterol lowering margarine in chapter eleven.

The Digestion and Absorption of Fat
This section will briefly describe what happens to the fat and cholesterol we eat once it enters our bodies. Nothing much happens to fat in our mouth and stomach, digestion of fat mostly occurs in the small intestines. The liver plays a major role in fat digestion because it produces bile, which is stored in the gallbladder and gets released into the small intestine after we have eaten a meal containing fat. Bile is actually produced largely from cholesterol and also contains bile salts and lecithin. Intestinal contractions mix the food we have eaten with bile, which emulsifies fat, or breaks it down into smaller droplets. Bile basically breaks fat molecules down into smaller pieces, so that fat digesting enzymes can work on it more effectively. People who have had their gallbladder taken out often find that a fatty meal will run straight through them, as they may not produce enough bile to break the fat down.

The pancreas makes a fat digesting enzyme, called lipase which works on digesting triglycerides, phospholipids and cholesterol in the small intestine. Phospholipids are a combination of fat and phosphate, and are the main component of cell membranes. Triglycerides, phospholipids and cholesterol are broken down into free fatty acids and other components, and absorbed into the mucosal cells that line the small intestine. The mucosal cells arrange the fat components into transport vehicles called chylomicrons. They are rich in triglycerides and transport fat to the lymphatic vessels, and then on to the liver and fat stores in the body. The liver makes various transport molecules for fats such as HDL, VLDL and LDL, which take fats to and from various body tissues.

The liver plays a very important role in regulating the fats in our bloodstream. It determines how much cholesterol it should produce by monitoring how much cholesterol is in the bloodstream. The more cholesterol you eat, the less your liver should manufacture, if it is healthy. Our liver acts like a filter, and helps to keep our bloodstream clean and prevents too much fat from accumulating in the bloodstream. In people with a fatty liver, this filter does not work efficiently; fatty tissue has been deposited in the liver, and excess fat accumulates in the bloodstream. This makes our blood cholesterol and triglyceride levels rise, and places us at increased risk of heart disease and strokes. A healthy liver removes excess fats from our body into bile, which then leaves our body through bowel motions.

Chapter Five

CORONARY HEART DISEASE

Coronary Heart Disease

You have probably heard this term many times, but do you really understand what it means? First we will describe the structure and function of a healthy heart.

Structure and Function of the Heart

The heart is a muscular pump located slightly to the left in the thoracic cavity. It is protected by the sternum, or breast bone and ribs, and is the shape of an inverted cone. An adult heart is approximately the size of a clenched fist and weighs about 340 grams (12 ounces). The heart and all the blood vessels of the body form the cardiovascular system. The main job of the heart is to pump blood through the blood vessels, so that it reaches all the organs and tissues of the body. Our heart circulates between five and six liters of blood around our body per minute, and around 13 liters per minute during vigorous exercise. Ref.25

The heart is divided into two sides, and each side has two chambers. Therefore, the heart contains four chambers: the left and right atrium at the top of the heart, and the left and right ventricles at the bottom of the heart. The right side of the heart receives oxygen deficient blood from the body, and pumps it into the lungs. The left side of the heart receives oxygen rich blood from the lungs, and pumps it out to the rest of the body through the aorta. The aorta is the largest blood vessel in the body. It has many branches that divide to supply blood to all areas of the body. The heart also needs its own blood supply; this is provided by the right and left coronary arteries, which are branches of the aorta.

The diagram below shows the different chambers of the heart, and the direction the blood travels in:

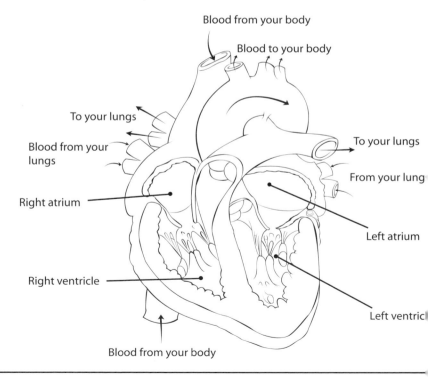

What is Coronary Heart Disease?

Also called coronary artery disease, this is the most common type of heart disease. The cause of coronary artery disease is atherosclerosis; whereby plaque builds up inside the arteries that supply the heart with blood. The plaque is made up of fat, cholesterol, calcium, smooth muscle cells, immune cells and other substances. You can read about atherosclerosis in more detail in chapter eight. As the plaque accumulates, less blood is able to reach the heart. Sometimes diminished blood flow to the heart causes chest pain, or angina.

A **heart attack** occurs when blood supply to the heart is severely reduced or stopped. Doctors refer to a heart attack as a myocardial infarction. The plaque that builds up in the arteries can eventually burst, tear or rupture, producing a blood clot that blocks the artery. If the blood supply stops for more than a few minutes, the muscle cells of the heart can be permanently injured and die. The heart attack can be fatal, depending on how much heart muscle has been damaged.

Sometimes there are no or very few symptoms to indicate that you are suffering from coronary artery disease. Symptoms are usually triggered by physical activity, stress, exposure to cold weather and sexual activity.

The most common symptoms of coronary heart disease are:

- Chest pain (this is usually a heavy, squeezing or crushing feeling)
- Neck, shoulder, arm, jaw or abdominal pain
- Weakness and shortness of breath
- Nausea with possible vomiting
- Perspiration

Symptoms are different in women

Recent studies have shown that the symptoms of heart disease are quite different in men and women. Only 30 percent of women who are proven to suffer with coronary heart disease experience any chest pain or chest distress. The most common symptoms of heart disease, experienced by 70 percent of affected women are unusual fatigue, sleep disturbance and shortness of breath. If women do experience an uncomfortable feeling in their chest, it is usually not as severe as in men. Ref 26.

Atherosclerosis is not the only possible cause of a heart attack. A coronary artery can contract, go into spasm and narrow, which also impairs blood flow to the heart. The exact cause of spasms is not known, however magnesium is very useful for helping to relax blood vessels.

Cerebrovascular disease is usually the result of plaque buildup in the arteries that supply the brain with blood. Cerebrovascular disease can cause a transient ischemic attack (TIA) or a stroke. A transient ischemic attack is where a person experiences a sudden loss of brain function but has a complete recovery within 24 hours. A hemorrhagic stroke is a different type of stroke where a blood vessel in the brain bursts.

Possible symptoms of a stroke or TIA include:

• Weakness or paralysis on one side of the body
• Jumbled speech and/or inability to comprehend speech
• Poor coordination
• Muscle weakness
• Loss of vision in one eye
• Paralysis of facial muscles
• Dizziness
• Rapid, involuntary eye movements

According to the medical community, the following are the major risk factors for coronary heart disease and cerebrovascular disease:

• Cigarette smoking
• High blood cholesterol
• Being overweight or obese
• Advancing age
• Male gender
• Family history of heart disease
• Stress

- Lack of exercise
- Diabetes

Chapter Six

DRUGS USED TO LOWER CHOLESTEROL: HOW THEY WORK & THEIR SIDE-EFFECTS

Drugs Used To Lower Cholesterol

In this section you will learn the major types of cholesterol lowering drugs, how they work, and the possible side effects they can have. If your doctor discovers that you have high blood levels of cholesterol and/or triglycerides, you will typically be given approximately six weeks to try and get your levels down through diet and exercise. The usual recommendation is to follow a low fat, high carbohydrate diet. This doesn't work for the majority of people since carbohydrates promote insulin release, which stimulates cholesterol production. The next recommendation is to take medication.

The major classes of cholesterol lowering drugs are:

STATINS

Drug names and brand names: Atorvastatin *(Lipitor)*, simvastatin *(Zocor)*, pravastatin *(Pravachol)*, lovastatin *(Mevacor, Altocor)*, fluvastatin *(Lescol, Lescol XL)*, Rosuvastatin *(Crestor)*.

How do statins work? These are the most widely prescribed lipid lowering drugs. In 1987 lovastatin became the first approved statin in the USA. These drugs inhibit the enzyme HMG-CoA reductase, which is responsible for producing cholesterol in the liver. Statins can lower cholesterol levels by 20-60% by reducing cholesterol production, and improving the liver's ability to get rid of LDL "bad" cholesterol from the bloodstream. Blood levels of triglycerides usually come down too. New research has shown that statin drugs may lower the risk of heart disease through a different mechanism than cholesterol reduction. Studies have shown that statins can lower blood levels of C-reactive protein (CRP); a marker of inflammation in the body, and a major risk factor for heart disease. You can read more about C-reactive protein in chapter eight. Statins are taken in the evening, as most cholesterol production occurs at night.

Side effects of statins: According to medical literature and the pamphlets inside the box of statins, they are well tolerated and side effects are rare; occurring in less than two percent of the population. The most common side effects are said to be constipation, flatulence, abdominal pain and indigestion. In reality, many people experience far worse side effects. More and more potential side effects are recently being discovered, exposing the fact that statins are not the wonder drugs they are marketed as.

How Statins Cause Side Effects

You may remember that cholesterol production begins with the molecule called acetyl-CoA. A number of metabolic reactions occur, until finally an enzyme called HMG-CoA reductase is required to convert a substance called HMG-CoA into mevalonate. Statins work by inhibiting the enzyme HMG-CoA reductase, thereby they inhibit mevalonate production. Mevalonate is a precursor to several substances, including cholesterol, sex hormones and adrenal hormones and Co Enzyme Q10. So as well as inhibiting cholesterol production, statins also inhibit the manufacture of many vital substances in our body.

Co Enzyme Q 10 (Co Q10) is also known as ubiquinone; it is formed in the mitochondria of each cell of our body, and is needed for energy production. Co Q10 is found in very high concentrations in cells that use a lot of energy, such as heart cells and skeletal muscle cells. It improves oxygen use by these cells, helping them to function. Co Enzyme Q 10 has many benefits for the heart, including:

- It is necessary for the production of collagen and elastin, helping to keep the blood vessels healthy.
- Acts as a strong antioxidant, protecting LDL "bad" cholesterol from oxidation.
- Reduces the risk of blood clots and rupture of fatty plaques in arteries.
- Needed for energy production by the heart and other cells.

Co Q 10 is considered one of the most important nutrients for a healthy heart, and yet statins deplete your body's production of it. Many of the side effects of statin drugs are probably caused by depletion of Co Q 10. Side effects of deficiency of this vital nutrient include:

- Muscle wasting, causing weakness and muscle pain.
- Heart failure (a deficiency weakens the heart muscle, making it less able to pump blood efficiently).
- Neuropathy (damage to the nervous system).
- Inflammation of the tendons and ligaments.

You are especially susceptible to suffer statin induced side effects if you are:
- Elderly
- Female
- Diabetic
- Postoperative

- If you have a liver or kidney disease
- If you take other medication, especially erythromycin, fibrates, itraconazole, or immunosuppressive drugs.

The following is a list of potential side effects of statin drugs:

- **Raised liver enzymes:** Statins can cause some inflammation and damage to your liver, thereby giving you raised liver enzymes. For this reason it is recommended that your doctor orders a blood test called a liver function test before you start taking a statin, and 12 weeks later. You are more likely to have raised liver enzymes if you take a statin along with another cholesterol lowering drug at the same time, such as Lopid (gemfibrozil) or niacin (vitamin B3) at high, prescription doses.

The irony is that many people who are put on statin drugs have a fatty liver and may already have raised liver enzymes. If you carry excess weight over your abdominal area, especially your upper abdomen, it is quite likely that you have a fatty liver. People with a fatty liver have an excessive amount of inflammation in their liver, and statin drugs will worsen this. Because the liver is the main site of cholesterol production, the reason your cholesterol is high is because your liver is dysfunctional. Taking a statin drug does nothing to improve your liver health, it does the opposite and worsens liver disease.

Therese in Western Australia has tried three different statins: Pravachol, Zocor and Lipitor. Therese recalled "All three drugs seem to raise my (liver) enzyme levels and now I have given up with feeling so lousy". She experienced "constant pain in my legs from the knee down, and a constant feeling of weakness in my calf muscles. I also feel nausea not long after taking the tablet".

- **Muscle soreness and weakness:** Statins can cause muscle pain and tenderness, called statin myopathy. The pharmaceutical industry claims that only two to three percent of people experience muscle pain, but reality may be quite different. Dr Beatrice Golomb, MD, Ph D from the University of California, San Diego, USA is conducting a study funded by the National Institute of Health on the side effects of statins. She has found that 98 percent of patients taking Lipitor suffer with muscle problems. Ref.27.

You are more likely to experience this side effect if you regularly exercise, as Co Enzyme Q10, which is depleted by statin drugs is needed for muscles to contract. People who take statins usually take a lot longer to recover from exercise than people who don't; they experience muscle pain for several days afterwards. Fibromyalgia is usually aggravated by statins also.

Statins are capable of causing a much more severe form of myopathy called **rhabdomyolysis**. This is where muscle cells break down and release a protein called myoglobulin into the bloodstream. Myoglobulin can impair kidney function and cause kidney failure, with eventual death. Certain medications increase the risk of developing rhabdomyolysis if taken with statins; these include:

- Fibrates (another type of cholesterol lowering drug)
- Erythromycin (an antibiotic)
- Antifungal medications
- Niacin at high, prescription doses
- Cyclosporine (an anti-rejection drug for patients who have had an organ donation).

You can have a blood test to see if statins are causing muscle damage; a substance called **creatine kinase (CK)** will be elevated. However, many people experience muscle pain and tenderness even if their creatine kinase levels are normal. Patients who experience muscle pain and muscle damage from statins may never fully recover; in some cases the myopathy is not reversible.

June from Victoria, in Australia could not tolerate statin drugs because of the myopathy they caused. According to June, "I stopped taking my cholesterol lowering medication (Zocor) because it made the muscles in the back of my legs so painful that I could not go for my morning walk."

Hal in the UK had a much worse experience. He was 32 years of age, with a diagnosed fatty liver and raised liver enzymes when his doctor put him on a low dose of Lipitor (10mg). It was after the first week of taking Lipitor that he started to experience "an unbelievable fatigue". According to Hal, "Walking became almost impossible, and if I did decide to walk to the end of the garden I had to crawl. My sister remarked that I had become an old man within a week". Hal immediately stopped taking Lipitor and decided to tackle his high cholesterol with diet and nutritional supplements. His liver enzymes are now normal, and his cholesterol is down to a healthy 206mg/dL.

• **Neuropathy:** Statins can cause nerve damage resulting in symptoms such as tingling, pain, numbness and weakness in the hands and feet. Some people even experience difficulty walking because of this. Researchers studied 500, 000 residents of Denmark and found that taking statins for one year raised the risk of nerve damage by 15 percent. People who took statins for two or more years were 26 percent more likely to get nerve damage. Ref.28 Cholesterol is a major component of the myelin sheath, which insulates our nerves and facilitates nerve transmissions.

Anne in NSW, Australia had been taking 40mg of Zocor (simvastatin) for 18 months before she noticed any side effects. Her cholesterol had been 246mg/dL and she couldn't get it down any lower with diet and exercise, so her doctor decided to put her on Zocor. The fact that Anne is a type 2 diabetic made her an even more suitable candidate for statin therapy according to her doctor. Anne has got a fatty liver, and her liver enzymes were elevated even before she started taking Zocor, yet her doctor still recommended she take it. Anne suffers with high blood pressure and takes Avapro 300, and has an under active thyroid, and takes Synthroid for this.

The first unusual symptoms Anne noticed were a feeling of nausea and what she described as "dead legs"; her legs felt extremely weak and heavy. She started sweating, developed pins and needles and felt overpoweringly ill. Anne assumed that she had come down with a virus. A week later her legs became even weaker and she noticed that her arms were trembling. The nerves in her arms and legs tingled and she felt like she was on the verge of suffering an anxiety attack, even though she had never experienced that before. Anne commented that her hands trembled as though she had Parkinson's disease.

Anne accidentally forgot to take Zocor for the next few days and started feeling better. She resumed the drug and the next morning felt incredibly weak, was trembling, shaking and sweating. The next thing she noticed, she could hardly stand. That was when Anne was taken to hospital. She underwent numerous tests which came up with nothing specific. Anne did not have an infection and her liver enzymes were still raised as previously. She was taken off Zocor, and then resumed it one last time, only to have all these symptoms return. Her doctors concluded that the only possible explanation for all of these symptoms was an adverse reaction to Zocor.

Anne was permanently taken off Zocor and the dose of her blood pressure tablet was reduced. It has now been one month since Anne discontinued Zocor, and she is slowly getting better. She used to walk 12 miles each week for exercise but cannot manage anything near this now; even going shopping is a strain on her legs. Anne still notices the occasional tremors in her hands.

The information leaflet inside a box of Zocor recommends it be used in people with diabetes, a history of stroke, or other blood vessel disease, regardless of their cholesterol level, in order to prolong their life. It is recommended that you do not take Zocor if you have a liver disease; Anne had a fatty liver yet she was still prescribed this medication. Paresthesia is listed as a possible side effect of Zocor, this is a nervous system disorder whereby people experience burning, prickling or stinging sensations. Anne experienced an extreme case of an adverse drug reaction. She has now been placed on an appropriate eating plan with nutritional supplements, and day by day she is slowly recovering her health.

- **Cancer:** In every study done on rodents, statins have caused cancer. A review published in the *Journal of the American Medical Association* states that *"All members of the two most popular classes of lipid-lowering drugs (the fibrates and the statins) cause cancer in rodents, in some cases at levels of animal exposure close to those prescribed to humans."* Ref 29. Studies done on humans have not produced such dramatic results because cancer is a disease that takes a long time to develop, and most clinical trials done on statins have not gone on for more than two or three years. This same study made the following final statement: *"the results of experiments in animals and humans suggest that lipid-lowering drug treatment, especially with the fibrates and statins, should be avoided except in patients at high short-term risk of coronary heart disease."* These studies have been conveniently forgotten, because millions of patients around the world are being put on cholesterol lowering drugs even if they have very few risk factors. Statins are also a drug that must be taken for life. One study done on humans, called the CARE trial found that breast cancer rates in those taking statins went up 1500 percent. Ref.30. Statins may get your cholesterol down, but at what price?

• **Heart Failure**: The world has experienced an enormous increase in the incidence of congestive heart failure. The incidence of heart attacks has gone down slightly, but heart failure rates are going up. After the age of 65, ten out of every 1000 people in the US develop congestive heart failure. Ref.31 Congestive heart failure occurs when the heart becomes weaker and cannot pump blood around the body as well as it should. Over time the heart becomes enlarged, thickened, and continues to get weaker. It becomes much less efficient at pumping blood.

Statins deplete the body of Co Enzyme Q10; the heart is a muscle, and heavily relies on Co Q 10 for energy. Without Co Q10, the mitochondria in the cells making up the heart cannot produce enough energy, leading to muscle weakness. The higher your dose of statins, and the longer you take them, the more likely you are to end up with heart failure. Ironically, virtually all patients with heart failure are placed on statins, supposedly to protect them against heart attacks, even if their cholesterol is normal.

• **Memory and concentration problems:** Statins may affect your cognitive function. A study done at the University of Pittsburgh in the USA showed that patients who took statins for six months performed much worse in solving complex mazes, memory tests, and had poorer psychomotor skills than patients who took a placebo.Ref.32 Lapses in concentration, and short term memory loss may not be just because you are tired or getting older, it could be the cholesterol lowering drug you are taking. Duane Graveline is a former astronaut and author of the book *"Lipitor: Thief of Memory"*. In his book Duane describes how he and many others have experienced complete memory loss for varying periods of time; they did not remember where they were and why. These memory blanks can occur suddenly and vanish suddenly. Lipitor (atorvastatin) and Zocor (simvastatin) are the statins most likely to cause memory loss. Ref.33

Cognitive decline is not mentioned as a possible side effect of statins in patient leaflets. In fact, some doctors actually recommend that taking statins, and having a low cholesterol level can help to prevent Alzheimer's disease. However, recent research disputes this. A group of 1026 individuals who were part of the Framingham study were observed. All the participants were free of cardiovascular disease and dementia in 1988-89, and had their cholesterol levels checked twice a year between 1950 and 2000. Between 1992 and 2000, 77 people developed Alzheimer's disease. The study found that the risk of developing Alzheimer's disease was in no way related to cholesterol levels. Ref.34

• **Depression:** Because cholesterol is required for the function of serotonin receptors in our brain, it makes sense that lowering cholesterol may trigger depression in some individuals. This is ironic, as depression is already a major health issue in the US, and people who are depressed are at greater risk of heart disease.

Mr R. C. from Albury in Australia experienced significant depression while taking Lipitor. "For the past 15 years I have been in a high stress position dealing with teenagers and young people in a country high school. About 3 years ago I had my cholesterol checked, and my G.P.

recommended I go onto Lipitor to lower the level of cholesterol. Over a period of time I began to feel depressed, wishing that there was some way out of the daily grind. I even took long service leave to see if the depression would lift, but it just kept getting stronger and stronger. I hated going to work. Once I was simply working on some landscaping at home when I broke down and cried on the front foot path. I wasn't even embarrassed about it. I couldn't care any more. There was no rhyme or reason for this apparent depression. I just felt awful and wanted to end my life.

Twelve months ago I had an appointment with Dr Cabot who asked what current medication I was taking. I listed several including Lipitor (the others were for high blood pressure) and she advised me to immediately stop taking the Lipitor.
The difference was very noticeable. I felt somewhat better during the next day when I didn't take the Lipitor and within a week I actually looked forward to going to work. Life has become a much happier place for me and I now look forward to a full and rewarding life. All the things that people do every day without thinking about I can now do with a positive outlook, and I am now living my life to the fullest".

Please note that we do not recommend you stop taking a cholesterol lowering medication abruptly, unless you have your own doctor's permission.

• **Ruined sex life:** Cholesterol is the building block for several hormones, including those made by the adrenal glands, as well as sex hormones. This means that taking cholesterol lowering drugs can lower testosterone levels in men and women, reducing libido, physical and mental drive, and energy. As well as a loss of sex drive, several studies have shown that cholesterol lowering drugs can affect sexual performance in men, leading to erectile dysfunction. This is the case for both statins and fibrates (another type of cholesterol lowering drug). Ref.35 Cells in the testes are capable of producing cholesterol, as it is required in high amounts to produce testosterone. Statin drugs do reach the testes, and they can inhibit cholesterol production there, as well as in the liver.

Ref.36. Sexual dysfunction symptoms vanish when the medications are discontinued.

The drug simvastatin (Zocor) is able to directly inhibit testosterone production independently of its cholesterol lowering action, via a different mechanism. Ref.37 In some men statin drugs have caused them to develop gynecomastia; this is the growth of breast tissue in men. The Australian Adverse Drug Reaction Advisory Committee has eleven reports of gynecomastia connected to simvastatin use. The UK Committee on Safety of Medicines lists "a few cases" of gynecomastia linked with the use of cholesterol lowering drugs. Ref.38

Be aware that the risk factors for coronary heart disease, such as obesity, diabetes and smoking are also risk factors for erectile dysfunction. If you do suffer with erectile dysfunction, it could be an early warning sign that you also have clogged arteries and are at risk of a heart attack or stroke.

• **Cataracts:** Taking statin drugs can cause irreversible damage to the lens of the eye. Taking the antibiotic erythromycin in combination with a statin increases the chances of developing cataracts. A study published in the *Archives of Internal Medicine* found that a single course of an antibiotic, typically lasting ten days doubled the risk of cataracts when taken with a statin. Two or more courses of antibiotics tripled the risk. Ref.39

Crestor: The latest but not the greatest

The newest statin on the market, released in September 2003 is called Crestor (rosuvastatin). It is made by the drug company AstraZeneca. Crestor has been clouded in controversy almost from the moment it was released. Dr Steven Galson, director of the FDA's center for drug evaluation and research has stated the FDA "has been very concerned about Crestor since the day it was approved, and we've been watching it very carefully".

Public Citizen, a health advocacy group has called for Crestor to be withdrawn due to an unacceptably high level of side effects. According to Public Citizen, there have been 29 reports of kidney failure or insufficiency in patients who took Crestor in its first year in the US. Considering that Crestor is not as commonly prescribed as the other types of statins, that was 75 times the rate of kidney failure or insufficiency of all similar drugs combined. Statin drugs can cause kidney failure through rhabdomyolysis; the breakdown of muscle cells which release substances that travel to the kidneys, and if severe enough can cause kidney failure.

Between October 1, 2003 and September 30, 2004 reports of rhabdomyolysis received by the FDA were 6.2 times higher for Crestor than all other statin drugs combined. Ref. 40   People with Asian ancestry are especially susceptible to the side effects of Crestor, as blood levels of this drug can rise to twice the level seen in Caucasian populations.

Are Statins Effective at Preventing Death?

There is so much emphasis on cholesterol, and trying to lower it, that the big picture has been lost. Cholesterol is over rated, and it isn't the huge risk factor for heart disease that the drug companies would like us to believe. It is excessive inflammation and oxidized cholesterol that cause harm to our heart and result in death. The ultimate goal is to lower the incidence of death from heart disease, not to lower a particular number. What is the point of having a low cholesterol level when the drugs you take to achieve this make you sick, and having low cholesterol puts you at risk of other diseases that can kill you or make your life miserable?

In order for a cholesterol lowering drug to be approved for sale by the FDA, a drug company must only prove that it lowers cholesterol levels; not necessarily that it reduces death from heart disease. Several long term studies have shown in patients taking statins, death rates from heart attacks do go down, but overall mortality stays the same for both groups. So the people who took statins died just as often as those who didn't, but from other causes. Statins reduce death from heart disease, but they usually don't reduce overall mortality.

If some Lipitor is good, more should be better?

A study published in the *New England Journal of Medicine*, called the TNT study analyzed 10 001 patients with established coronary heart disease (CHD) and an LDL "bad" cholesterol level less than 130mg/dL. The purpose of the study was to find out if getting LDL cholesterol below currently recommended levels offers any benefits to patients with coronary heart disease. The study aimed to lower LDL cholesterol levels below 100mg/dL.

The participants were divided into two groups; one group was given 10mg of atorvastatin (Lipitor), and the other received 80mg per day. The patients were followed for 4.9 years. Patients who took 80mg Lipitor got their LDL cholesterol down to an average of 77mg/dL, and those who took 10mg had a mean LDL of 101mg/dL. The incidence of liver problems (raised liver enzymes) was six times higher in the group given 80mg of Lipitor. The total deaths due to cardiovascular causes were 126 in the 80mg group, and 155 in the 10mg group. However, the total deaths due to other causes was 158 in the 80mg group, and 127 in the 10mg group. Ref.41. This means that more people died in the group taking a bigger dose of Lipitor! Clearly, if deaths due to coronary heart disease went down, but total deaths didn't, some other cause of death had to increase. Cancer accounted for more than half the deaths from non-cardiovascular causes in both groups of participants. However, the conclusion of this study did not mention that; it states that *"intensive lipid-lowering therapy with 80mg atorvastatin (Lipitor) per day in patients with stable CHD provides significant clinical benefit beyond that afforded by treatment with 10mg atorvastatin per day"*. This study was funded by Pfizer (the drug company that makes Lipitor), and conducted by Pfizer sponsored scientists. There was no control group in this study; no group was given a placebo. The authors of the study stated that it would be unethical to have a placebo group, as it would deny people of the benefits of Lipitor!

Do statins work in women?

So far there have not been any studies to show that statin drugs reduce death rates from heart disease in women. The University of British

Columbia Therapeutics Initiative has stated that statins offer no benefit to women for the prevention of heart disease. Ref.42. Yet more and more women are being put on these drugs, and women are more likely than men to experience their negative side effects. In the vast majority of controlled, randomized clinical trials done on statins, there has been no improvement in survival rates in women.

According to Dr James M. Wright, PhD, of the University of British Columbia, "combined results of all trials do not support the use of statins by women without heart disease". High blood cholesterol has never proven to be a risk factor for heart disease in women. At every age, women usually have higher blood cholesterol levels than men of the same age, yet women are around 15 years older than men when they have their first heart attack. The General Accounting Office of the US Government has recognized the lack of thorough clinical trials by stating *"the trials generally have not evaluated the efficacy of cholesterol-lowering treatment for several important population groups, such as women, elderly men and women, and minority men and women. Thus, they provide little or no evidence of benefits or possible risks for these groups"*.

As well as not reducing the risk of heart disease, statins can increase the risk of cancer. Three clinical trials have shown women who take statin drugs to have higher rates of breast cancer. In one trial, people with heart disease took 40mg of Pravachol (pravastatin) or a placebo daily. The study found that 12 out of 286 women taking Pravachol developed breast cancer, and only one out of 290 taking the placebo did. Ref.43 This result is claimed to be "not statistically significant", so you don't hear about it. Only the positive results are published because much of the research is funded by the company that makes the drug. Medical research is extremely expensive to carry out, therefore the drug companies have to make sure they recoup their money.

Are statins beneficial for older people?
For a start it is controversial whether high cholesterol is a problem in people over 70 years of age. A study called "Cholesterol and mortality:

30 years of follow-up from the Framingham study" was published in the *Journal of the American Medical Association* in 1987. Cholesterol levels were measured in 1959 men and 2415 women aged between 31 and 65 years of age, who were free of cardiovascular disease and cancer. You may be shocked to know that the study showed there was no increased death rate in people with high cholesterol over the age of 50. So if you make it to 50 years of age, you are not more likely to die of a heart attack if you have high cholesterol than people who have normal or low cholesterol, according to this study. In the study there was a direct association between low levels of cholesterol and increased death. Ref.44

Researchers at the San Diego School of Medicine found that high cholesterol in people over 75 years of age is protective, instead of harmful. They also stated that low cholesterol is a risk factor for heart arrhythmias, or heart rhythm irregularities. Ref.45 A study in the *European Heart Journal* recruited 595 people with coronary heart disease who had a total cholesterol level of 160mg/dL or less; they were compared with a group of 10 968 people with heart disease who had a cholesterol level above 160mg/dL. The study found that the risk of cardiac death was the same in both groups. Therefore, there was no protective benefit to having a low cholesterol level. The study found that *"the most frequent cause of non-cardiac death associated with low total cholesterol was cancer"*. Ref.46 What is the point of worrying about getting your cholesterol down when it won't help you to live any longer? Elderly patients are more susceptible to side effects caused by statin drugs. One reason for this is that older people are more likely to take several medications, making drug interactions more likely to happen. Statin induced muscle soreness (myopathy) is more common as we get older, the more other medications we take, the more other diseases we have, and during postoperative periods. All of these factors are more prevalent in the elderly. Muscle pain makes people less likely to exercise; therefore they miss out on the cardiovascular benefits it provides.

Statins without a prescription
In 2004 a low dose version of the cholesterol lowering drug Zocor became available without a prescription in the UK. The theory behind

this move was to make statins more widely available to the public, in order to prevent heart disease in at risk individuals. Dr John Reckless, chairman of Heart UK believes statins are safer than aspirin, and "rather more people do need statins than are currently getting them".

Statins can of course have serious side effects, and this move will place an unnecessarily high number of people at risk. They should never be used by pregnant women because they can cause limb defects. Professor Tom Sanders is a nutritionist at King's College, London, and nutrition director for Heart UK. According to Professor Sanders, "At the age of 40, your risk of having a heart attack is below one in 1, 000, so any reduction is really quite miniscule in terms of benefit". Ref.47 Unfortunately, being able to buy Zocor over the counter reinforces the idea that we can eat what we like and never exercise, and a pill will undo the damage.

The Story of Baycol

Baycol was a statin drug manufactured by the German drug company Bayer AG. It was approved for use in the United States by the FDA in 1997. On 8th August 2001 Bayer AG voluntarily withdrew the drug from the market because it was responsible for the deaths of 31 people in the USA. These people developed rhabdomyolysis which is a severe breakdown of muscle cells that causes muscle pain, weakness, tenderness, fever, dark urine, nausea and vomiting. Most people die of kidney failure when this happens. Rhabdomyolysis is a possible side effect of all cholesterol lowering drugs called statins. In one third of these cases, the victim was also taking another cholesterol lowering drug called gemfibrozil, which is known to increase the risk of this condition. Following the withdrawal, the FDA did not undertake any regulatory action with regard to the other cholesterol lowering drugs in the same category as Baycol.

Baycol was the third best selling prescription drug for Bayer, and in the year 2000 it earned the company $US 560 million in sales. It is very sad that people had to die when cholesterol levels can be normalized in most cases with an appropriate eating plan and improving liver function.

Between 1981 and 2000 the FDA approved 543 new drugs in the US. Fourteen of these drugs were subsequently recalled because of safety concerns. Ref.48. The drug Vioxx was withdrawn from the market in September 2004 because it was found to significantly increase the risk of heart attack and stroke. Why put your life in the hands of drug companies when nutritional medicine can prolong your life and improve its quality?

Are there any benefits to taking statins?

Some very recent studies are showing that statin drugs can reduce inflammation in the body; specifically they are able to lower C-reactive protein (CRP) levels. According to Dr Christopher P. Cannon, a cardiologist at Brigham and Women's Hospital in Boston, USA, "CRP is a global screen for bad things in the cardiovascular system". If you have high blood levels of this substance, you are much more likely to have a heart attack.

Currently the mechanism by which statin drugs lower CRP is not known, but patients who have low levels (especially lower then 2mg/L) are less likely to have a heart attack, regardless of what their LDL level is. Ref.49. Perhaps statin drugs are exerting their protective effects on cardiovascular disease not by lowering cholesterol, but by lowering C-reactive protein.

It is good to know that statins can do something useful for your health, like lowering inflammation, but there may be a high price to pay. It is very easy to lower C-reactive protein with a healthy diet and lifestyle. Maintaining a healthy weight, exercising regularly, and having a high intake of vegetable juices and antioxidants are simple ways to lower your CRP level. The thing is that these natural treatments don't make much money. Drug companies make enormous profits on cholesterol lowering drugs.

Other Types of Cholesterol Lowering Medications

BILE ACID SEQUESTRANTS

Drug names and brand names: Cholestyramine *(Questran Lite, Questran, Cholestyramine Light, Locholest, Locholest Light, Prevalite)*, colestipol *(Colestid, Cholestid Flavored)*.

How do bile acid sequestrants work? They bind with cholesterol containing bile acids in the intestines, and are then removed in bowel motions. These drugs typically lower LDL cholesterol by 10-20%. Sometimes a bile acid sequestrant is given with a statin drug in order to lower cholesterol levels more efficiently. Together, these two drugs can lower LDL cholesterol by approximately 40%. Triglycerides are not lowered by bile acid sequestrants. These drugs usually come as powders and are mixed with water or juice and consumed once or twice daily with meals.

Side effects of bile acid sequestrants: These drugs reduce your ability to absorb other medications you take. They also inhibit the absorption of the fat soluble vitamins A, E, D and K, therefore long term use of bile acid sequestrants usually requires vitamin supplementation. Antacids impair the effectiveness of bile acid sequestrants, therefore the two drugs should not be taken together. The most common side effects of these medications are digestive upsets such as gas, nausea, bloating and constipation.

CHOLESTEROL ABSORPTION INHIBITORS

Drug name and brand name: Ezetimibe *(Zetia)*.

How do cholesterol absorption inhibitors work? This is a new class of drugs which was first approved by the US FDA in late 2002. Ezetimibe inhibits the intestinal absorption of cholesterol found in bile and the diet. When given by itself, ezetimibe reduces LDL cholesterol by 18-20%. It is often given with a statin, especially in people who get side effects from high doses of statins. Ezetimibe can increase HDL cholesterol, but the way it does this is not yet known. It has no effect on the absorption of triglycerides, bile acids, fatty acids and fat soluble vitamins. This drug is taken in tablet form once daily.

Side effects of cholesterol absorption inhibitors: So far studies have shown that side effects in people taking ezetimibe were no greater than those taking a placebo. It is generally well tolerated if taken on its own.

NICOTINIC ACID AGENTS
Drug name and brand name: Niacin, nicotinic acid.

How do nicotinic acid agents work? Nicotinic acid is vitamin B3; a water soluble vitamin. When given in doses much higher than required for good health, niacin is able to lower LDL cholesterol and triglyceride levels, and raise HDL cholesterol levels. A typical starting dose is 250mg three times daily, which is usually increased up to a maximum daily dose of 3-4.5g. The Recommended Daily Intake (RDI) for niacin is only 13mg for women and 19mg for men. Nicotinic acid can lower LDL cholesterol by 10-20%, lower triglycerides by 20-50% and increase HDL cholesterol by 15-35%.

Side effects of nicotinic acid agents: The most common and annoying side effect is hot flashes, as it has the effect of dilating blood vessels. Clearly this is not the drug of choice for menopausal women! Digestive upsets such as nausea, indigestion, gas and diarrhea can occur. Nicotinic acid is contraindicated in people with peptic ulcers, as it can severely aggravate them. This drug can also enhance the effect of high blood pressure medication. Other problematic side effects include gout, an increase in blood sugar levels and inflammation of the liver.

FIBRATES

Drug names and brand names: Gemfibrozil *(Lopid)*, fenofibrate *(Antara, Tricor)*.

How do fibrates work? The exact mechanism is not fully understood; however fibrates do lower triglyceride and VLDL levels, and can slightly increase HDL cholesterol levels. These drugs come in tablet and capsule form, and are typically taken twice daily, half an hour before the morning and evening meals.

Side effects of fibrates: The most common problem is gastrointestinal discomfort, and these drugs can increase the chance of developing gallstones. Fibrates can increase the effects of some drugs, making it more likely for you to suffer side effects from them; these drugs include the blood thinning drug Warfarin, some diabetic medications and statin drugs. If fibrates are taken together with statins, they greatly increase the chances of suffering severe side effects of statins such as myopathy (muscle pain), and rhabdomyolysis (the breakdown of muscle tissue). However, the medical profession does recommend these two drugs are combined in high risk people if one drug has not worked on its own. Regular blood tests for liver enzymes and creatine kinase (CK) are recommended if statins and fibrates are taken together to monitor side effects.

PROBUCHOL

This is not a commonly used drug because it lowers both the LDL "bad" and HDL "good" cholesterol. Therefore, it is only used in some types of hereditary high cholesterol cases or in patients where other cholesterol lowering drugs have been ineffective. Probuchol can cause nausea, bloating, diarrhea and dizziness.

Chapter Seven

THE HAZARDS OF LOW CHOLESTEROL

Many people believe that they will be healthier, and live a longer life if they can get their cholesterol as low as possible. Drug companies would have us believe that the lower we can get our cholesterol levels the better. This is false and is no more than a plot to sell more cholesterol lowering drugs. You may remember from chapter one that cholesterol has a lot of important functions in our body. When we don't have enough of it, either through the use of medication, strict dieting, or having naturally low levels, several health problems can arise.

The following are health conditions that have all been linked to too low cholesterol:

AGGRESSIVE BEHAVIOR, DEPRESSION AND SUICIDE

Cholesterol is needed for the serotonin receptors in the brain to function. Serotonin is the "feel good" chemical in our brain that helps to keep our mood stable, and makes us feel happy. Popular antidepressant medications such as Prozac, Zoloft and Celexa are called Selective Serotonin Reuptake Inhibitors (SSRIs) because they work to keep the levels of serotonin in our brain high. Epidemiological studies have linked low cholesterol levels with increased rates of mortality due to suicide, violence and accidents. Ref.50, 51

Studies have also shown that people with low cholesterol levels have lower levels of serotonin. Dutch researchers measured the cholesterol levels of 30, 000 men and compared the incidence of depression, anger, impulsivity and hostility in these men with their incidence in men with normal cholesterol levels. They discovered that men with chronically low cholesterol have a higher incidence of depression and related symptoms. Ref.52. Some patients experience irritability and a short temper while taking cholesterol lowering medication, which resolves when they discontinue it. One study found that school aged children with a cholesterol level below 144mg/dL were almost three times more likely to be expelled or suspended from school than children with higher cholesterol levels. Ref.53

SLOWER BRAIN FUNCTION

Cholesterol is a major component of our brain. Our nerve cells are insulated by a fatty material called myelin. You may have heard of myelin, as it is the substance that is destroyed in the disease multiple sclerosis. Myelin is made up of 70 percent fat; 28 percent of which is cholesterol. Ref.54 The high cholesterol content allows myelin to wrap tightly around nerve cells, speeding messages through the brain. This is probably why having a too low cholesterol level slows your brain down. A study was conducted by Professor Michael Muldoon, as part of the third National Health and Nutrition Examination Survey. The relationship between blood cholesterol and cognitive performance was tested in over four thousand people. It was discovered that lower blood cholesterol levels in men correlated with slower visuomotor speed; this is a measure of how quickly you react in emergency situations. Ref.55

WEAK IMMUNE SYSTEM

Having a low cholesterol level makes you more susceptible to infections, especially post operative infections. Ref.56. Hospitalized patients with low cholesterol are more likely to die than patients who have normal or high cholesterol levels. Ref.57 The lipoproteins that carry cholesterol around our bloodstream help to protect us against the harmful effects of bacterial endotoxins, which are released whenever we have a bacterial infection. Ref.58t. Since cholesterol is a fat, it helps to carry the antioxidant, fat soluble vitamins E and A around our body.

People with high cholesterol have stronger immune systems than people with low cholesterol; they have greater numbers of various immune cells. Clearly you need some cholesterol in your body to help keep your immune system strong.

HORMONE DEFICIENCIES

The sex hormones estrogen, progesterone, testosterone and DHEA, as well as the adrenal hormones aldosterone and cortisol are all referred to as steroid hormones. All of these hormones are made in the body from cholesterol. If you did not have cholesterol in your body, you would not be able to make any of these hormones.

The diagram below describes how cholesterol is converted into the various steroid hormones.

How cholesterol is converted into steroid hormones

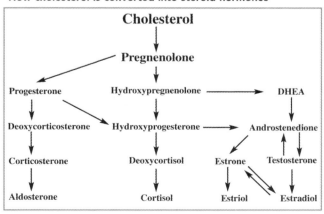

The parent molecule from which all steroid hormones are manufactured is called pregnenalone. This is an important hormone, as it helps to prevent inflammatory conditions such as arthritis, eczema, fibromyalgia and auto-immune conditions. Cortisol is an anti-inflammatory hormone produced by the adrenal glands, and it is involved in the metabolism of carbohydrate and protein. Aldosterone is another adrenal hormone that controls water and sodium balance in the kidneys.

Many people who take cholesterol lowering medication experience a reduction in their libido; this makes sense as their body is less able to produce sex hormones. Low levels of sex hormones may also contribute to erectile dysfunction and aggravate the symptoms of fibromyalgia, such as aching, tender muscles.

SHORTER LIFE SPAN

People with low cholesterol die earlier than those with normal to high levels, and they seem to have higher rates of cancer. A study titled "Low serum total cholesterol is associated with marked increase in mortality in advanced heart failure" was published in the *Journal of Cardiac Failure*. 1 134 patients were studied, and low cholesterol was associated with worse outcomes and impaired survival in patients with heart failure. People with higher cholesterol had better survival rates. In this study, the researchers observed that high cholesterol in these patients was not associated with high blood pressure, diabetes or coronary heart disease. Ref.60

A study of 4 521 Italian men and women between the ages of 65 and 84 was published in the *Journal of the American Geriatrics Society*. The study found that people with a total cholesterol level below 187mg/dL are at higher risk of dying, even when many other factors are taken into account. Low cholesterol levels seem to be associated with poor health, or declining health.

GREATER RISK OF CANCER

It has long been noted that people with low levels of cholesterol are more likely to develop cancer than people with normal or high levels. This pattern occurs among all age groups. Austrian researchers followed more than 149, 000 women and men (aged 20-95 years) for 15 years as part of the European Health Monitoring and Promotion Programme. Low cholesterol was found to be a significant risk factor for all-cause mortality in men across the entire age group, and in women, especially from the age of 50 onwards. People with low cholesterol suffered significantly more death from cancer, liver diseases and mental disorders. Ref.59

How Low Should You Go?

You should aim for a cholesterol level of 183mg/dL to 214mg/dL. Levels below 179mg/dL can be unhealthy. The all-cause death rate is higher in individuals with cholesterol levels lower than 179mg/dL. Ref.61

Chapter Eight

INFLAMMATION AND ITS ROLE IN HEART DISEASE

You may think that atherosclerosis is just a disease whereby fat accumulates on the inner lining of your arteries. The more fat you eat, the more fat accumulates inside your arteries and the greater your chances of having a heart attack. This was what the medical community believed for many years, and it is still what the majority of the public believes. This is a very simplistic view, and we now know that atherosclerosis is a much more complex process.

Scientists have discovered that inflammation is involved in every stage of atherosclerosis, from the beginning when a fatty streak develops, right through to the end when the fatty plaque breaks off and causes a blood clot which blocks blood flow in an artery, causing a heart attack. Inflammation is the way our body responds to injury. We can usually tell a part of our body is inflamed when it is red, hot, swollen and we can't move it properly. Think of a stubbed toe or a sprained ankle. Inflammation is present in all "itis" conditions, such as arthritis, hepatitis, bursitis, and many others. It is a normal reaction by our immune system to infection or injury. However, inflammation can also occur inside our body in a much more silent way, where we don't even know it is happening.

Inflammation can trigger the release of substances into our bloodstream that damage the inner lining of arteries. Cholesterol in the bloodstream can then put a protective coating over this damage. Cholesterol has a healing, protective quality; large amounts of it are present in scar tissue. As the damage to our arteries gets worse, more cholesterol accumulates, the fatty plaque grows and our arteries narrow.

C-Reactive Protein

This is a kind of protein that both promotes and reflects inflammation levels in our body. It is elevated in the bloodstream in a number of varied diseases. New research has shown that elevated blood levels of C-reactive protein (CRP) are a major risk factor for heart disease, possibly being more significant than cholesterol levels. CRP is an independent marker for future cardiovascular disease, meaning even if you have a low or normal cholesterol level, you are at great risk of heart disease if you have high CRP levels. Your doctor can easily order a blood test to check you CRP level; you can read more about blood tests in chapter ten.

The New England Journal of Medicine published an article stating that inflammation is a better indicator of who will have a heart attack than high cholesterol. In this study almost 28 000 healthy postmenopausal women had blood tests and were monitored for eight years. The women with high levels of CRP were twice as likely to have a heart attack or stroke as the women with high levels of LDL "bad" cholesterol! Ref.62 A study done on men published in the same journal showed that men with the highest CRP levels had three times the number of heart attacks and two times the amount of ischemic strokes as men with normal levels. The really interesting fact is that the incidence was independent of other risk factors including blood fat levels and smoking!

The theory is that having high CRP levels means you have chronic inflammation in the walls of your coronary arteries. This inflammation makes it more likely that fatty particles and immune cells will be attracted to the artery wall in an effort to repair the damage. This sets the stage for the development of a fatty plaque and full blown atherosclerosis. High blood levels of CRP indicate that you are more likely to have a heart attack, and the higher your level, the less likely you are to survive that heart attack. Recent studies have also shown that high CRP levels increase the chance of an artery re-closing after it has been opened by balloon angioplasty. Ref.63

What causes elevated C-reactive protein?

The following conditions are most likely responsible for high CRP:

- Chronic or acute infections.

- Autoimmune disease.

- Allergies.

- Obesity.

- Diabetes mellitus.

- Consuming trans fatty acids (hydrogenated vegetable oil) and oils high in omega 6 fats, such as soybean, corn, safflower, cottonseed and sunflower oils.

- Diets high in sugar, refined carbohydrates and high glycemic foods, such as white bread, potatoes, biscuits and breakfast cereals.

- Cigarette smoking.

- Lack of antioxidant nutrients in the diet.

Homocysteine

Homocysteine is an amino acid that forms in our body as a result of breakdown of dietary protein. It is also an intermediate molecule in the synthesis of the amino acid cysteine from methionine, (another amino acid). The main role of methionine in the body is to provide methyl groups for metabolic processes to occur. When methionine loses a methyl group it becomes homocysteine. In order for homocysteine to be converted back into methionine, it must receive a methyl group from either folic acid (vitamin B9), or vitamin B6. Vitamin B12 is needed as a co-factor for this reaction to occur.

Homocysteine can be measured in our bloodstream; a high reading usually indicates we do not get enough vitamins B6, B12 or folic acid in our diet. These vitamins are found in high amounts in fresh fruit and vegetables, as well as animal protein such as red meat, eggs and fish. Betaine is another nutrient helpful in keeping homocysteine low; it is found in high amounts in eggs. Diets high in processed foods are often lacking these nutrients. Having high blood levels of homocysteine is thought to be a major risk factor for heart disease, and several other diseases.

The inner lining of our arteries is called the endothelium. In healthy arteries the endothelial cells form a continuous protective layer, regulating which substances can pass from the bloodstream into the deeper artery wall. If our endothelial cells are injured and inflamed, it makes the artery lining more permeable, allowing molecules to enter the artery wall. Homocysteine has an abrasive action; it scrapes the inner lining of our blood vessels. People with high homocysteine levels have greater damage to the lining of their arteries and more atherosclerotic plaques. Ref.64. High levels of homocysteine also seem to activate platelets and increase the tendency for clots to form. A study published in the *Journal of the American Medical Association* showed that men with the highest homocysteine levels are three times more likely to have a heart attack, regardless of their cholesterol or triglyceride levels. Ref.65 High blood homocysteine levels have also been strongly linked with the following diseases: Alzheimer's disease, osteoporosis, depression, diabetes, multiple sclerosis, rheumatoid arthritis and birth defects. Ref.66

What Causes Elevated Homocysteine?

- Inadequate intake of folic acid, vitamin B6 or vitamin B12 in your diet, or malabsorption of these.

- Genetics. Some people have a genetic defect which affects their ability to absorb and use folic acid. These people need higher amounts of folic acid than a normal diet can provide, and they are best off taking a supplement.

- Stress. Adrenaline and noradrenaline are stress hormones and their metabolism requires methylation. This increases our need for vitamins B6, B12 and folic acid. If our intake is inadequate, homocysteine will build up.

- Coffee consumption. The more coffee we drink, the higher our homocysteine tends to be.

- Oral contraceptive use. This is because oral contraceptives deplete the body of vitamin B6 and folic acid. This may be one reason why oral contraceptives can increase the risk of heart disease.

- Impaired kidney function.

Atherosclerosis: What Really Happens to Our Arteries?

Atherosclerosis is a slow disease where fatty substances, cholesterol, calcium, various types of cells and other substances accumulate in the inner lining of arteries. These substances combine together to form a plaque on the artery. The word atherosclerosis is derived from the Greek words *athero* (meaning paste, or gruel), and *sclerosis* (meaning hardness). This process often begins in childhood and can become quite advanced by as early as age 25. Ref.67   Atherosclerosis will affect you differently depending on which arteries become clogged with fat; plaque buildup in arteries that supply the heart can lead to angina or a heart attack, and plaque buildup in arteries that supply the brain can lead to a stroke or transient ischemic attack. Ischemia means lack of oxygen, usually because of reduced blood supply. You will not notice any symptoms of atherosclerosis until approximately 40 percent of a blood vessel becomes obstructed.

Atherosclerosis is believed to be caused by damage to the innermost lining of an artery, called the endothelium. Several things can cause the damage, including high blood pressure, cigarette smoking, homocysteine, LDL "bad" cholesterol, diabetes, infections, and other factors that promote inflammation in the body. These are the real risk factors for heart disease and will be discussed in greater detail below. If the endothelium becomes damaged, it is easier for substances such as cholesterol, calcium and immune cells to be deposited inside the artery wall. This thickens the artery, therefore its diameter shrinks, blood flow diminishes and oxygen supply is greatly reduced. Cholesterol has a role in repair and healing. Scar tissue has a lot of cholesterol in it. If our artery wall becomes damaged, cholesterol circulating in the bloodstream clings to it, and over time can form a thick coating or plaque. Eventually the plaque can rupture, or a blood clot can form on top of the plaque, thereby completely blocking off the blood supply. The aim then is to avoid damage occurring to your artery wall in the first place. Cholesterol does not deposit itself on healthy, smooth blood vessels.

It all starts with inflammation

When there is too much inflammation in the body, the inner lining (endothelium) of the artery walls can become damaged. This causes the endothelial cells to produce various adhesion molecules that attract white blood cells and cause them to bind to the artery wall. The particular white blood cells that bind are monocytes and T lymphocytes. These blood cells migrate deep into the lining of the arteries. The monocytes turn into macrophages, which are a type of white blood cell that act like Pac man; they engulf dead cells, bacteria and various debris. The macrophages start ingesting LDL cholesterol, and once they are filled with fat, they are referred to as foam cells. It is especially oxidized LDL particles that are ingested; these are particles that have been damaged by free radicals, either because of the way food has been processed, or because we do not have enough antioxidants in our body to prevent this. Oxidized LDL cholesterol also causes direct damage to the endothelium.

Inflammatory chemicals called cytokines are produced by the white blood cells that have entered the artery wall. These cytokines attract more white blood cells to the area and also stimulate the growth of smooth muscle cells of the artery wall. As smooth muscle cells accumulate, they cause the artery wall to thicken, which narrows the diameter of the artery. The smooth muscle cells produce enzymes that cause the breakdown of collagen and elastin in the artery wall. The macrophages also produce protein digesting enzymes that break down collagen. This makes the fatty plaque unstable and prone to rupture. If it ruptures it is more likely to form a clot and block an artery completely. As atherosclerotic plaques progress, they tend to calcify, or harden because they accumulate calcium; this hardening is referred to as arteriosclerosis.

Damage to the endothelium also impairs the production of nitric oxide by cells lining the artery wall. Nitric oxide is your artery's best friend because it dilates the arteries, has an anti inflammatory effect, and limits the ability of white blood cells to bind to the artery wall and initiate plaque formation. Ref.68

Chapter Nine

WHAT CAUSES EXCESSIVE INFLAMMATION? THE REAL RISK FACTORS FOR HEART DISEASE

We now know that inflammation seems to be the trigger for atherosclerotic plaques to develop, progress and eventually rupture, but what causes the inflammation in the first place? In this chapter we will look at the various causes of inflammation in the body; these are the real risk factors for heart disease.

What Causes Inflammation?

• Obesity

Fat cells (adipocytes) do not just sit there and wobble, they actually produce a lot of hormones and inflammatory chemicals; the more fat cells we have, the more of these chemicals will be made. Fat cells manufacture and secrete biologically active messenger molecules called cytokines. These cytokines are thought to greatly increase the risk of developing heart disease because they can irritate and damage the artery walls. Some of the chemical messengers produced by fat cells include leptin, adiponectin, plasminogen activator inhibitor-1, resistin, interleukin-6, adipsin and tumor necrosis factor; each of these can have destructive effects if produced in excess. Ref.69

Being overweight works against you in two ways; fat cells secrete chemicals that promote inflammation in your body, and the inflammatory chemicals promote the formation of more fat cells, causing you to gain more weight. Overweight people usually have higher amounts of C-reactive protein in their bloodstream.

As well as increasing systemic inflammation and promoting the development of atherosclerosis, chemicals made by fat cells have effects on fat and blood sugar metabolism. Some of these substances make it harder for insulin to work in our body, thus having too much fat on our body can cause Syndrome X and diabetes. Researchers at the University of Buffalo have shown that two types of white blood cells, monocytes and lymphocytes are in a much more active state in obese people. These cells enter the artery wall and start the process of atherosclerosis, they activate fat cells to produce more inflammatory cytokines, and they interfere with insulin function, causing Syndrome X. Ref.70. C-reactive protein is mainly produced in the liver; if you have a fatty liver, your liver cells produce more inflammatory cytokines which then stimulate your liver to make more C-reactive protein. Ref.71

Fat cells can even produce chemicals that cause constriction of blood vessels and raise your blood pressure. Fat stores in the abdominal area secrete inflammatory chemicals that go straight to the liver and inflame it. This causes raised liver enzymes and the development of fatty liver disease. In overweight people, large amounts of free fatty acids travel from the fat stores to the liver where they stimulate the production of VLDL cholesterol. This is the worst kind of cholesterol, as it is rich in triglycerides. The high levels of VLDL suppress the production of HDL "good" cholesterol.

Clearly losing weight is one of the best ways to lower the amount of inflammation in your body, and in that way reduce your chances of developing heart disease and diabetes.

• Oxidized Fatty Acids and Cholesterol
Many researchers believe that cholesterol itself does not cause heart disease, but rather oxidized cholesterol is to blame. Fats become oxidized when they are exposed to light, oxygen or heat. Because of our typical processed food diets, most people ingest a great deal of oxidized fats.

When unsaturated fatty acids (mostly found in vegetable oil) are refined and processed in their manufacture, much of these fats become oxidized. If we eat food that has been fried or deep fried in these fats, we are consuming a great deal of toxic oxidation products formed in these oils. The intense heat used for frying creates compounds including peroxides, hydroperoxides, ozonides, polymers and hydroperoxyaldehydes. These dangerous compounds inflame and irritate your artery walls, damage cell membranes and impair your immune function. They also have the ability to irritate your liver cells and start the development of fatty liver disease. Whenever you eat food that has been fried in vegetable oil, you will be taking in toxic compounds that create a lot of free radical damage in your body. Extra virgin olive oil and virgin coconut fat are exceptions to this rule.

Oxidized cholesterol is found in foods like processed deli meats, foods containing powdered eggs and powdered milk, and egg yolks if the eggs have been cooked in a way that the yolk is broken and heated to high temperatures, for example frying. Homogenized milk is more likely to contain oxidized cholesterol than un-homogenized milk, because the fat globules are smaller, and thus have a greater surface area. This leaves them more susceptible to damage by light, oxygen and heat.

Fatty acids and cholesterol can be oxidized in our own bodies too. We may eat fresh, unrefined fats, but if our body is lacking antioxidants, these fats can still become damaged. Anything that increases the amount of free radicals in our body makes us more susceptible to fat oxidation; these factors include stress, lack of sleep, exposure to pollution, ultraviolet radiation from the sun and a diet lacking raw vegetables and fruit.

If we ingest, or otherwise form oxidized cholesterol in our body, this cholesterol will be incorporated into our lipoproteins; HDL, LDL and others. We know that LDL is the "bad" kind of cholesterol, but when it becomes oxidized it is so much worse. It is believed that oxidized LDL causes much more damage to artery walls because it is able to stick to the artery walls much more readily. Lecithin helps to protect cholesterol from oxidation; it is found in high amounts in eggs and soy foods.

• Diabetes

Diabetes is probably the biggest risk factor for heart disease. More than 50 percent of people with type 2 diabetes die of coronary artery disease. Ref.72 Usually women are protected from cardiovascular disease somewhat before they reach menopause, however women with type 2 diabetes are just as susceptible to heart disease as men. Ref.73. Diabetics are less likely to survive a heart attack than non-diabetics.

In diabetics all of the risk factors associated with being overweight are magnified. Most diabetics are overweight, and their fat stores produce large amounts of inflammatory cytokines. The arteries of diabetics are not able to produce adequate levels of nitric oxide, which acts to dilate blood vessels and reduce inflammation. The artery walls of diabetics also produce more free radicals, which further worsen inflammation and promote the oxidation of LDL cholesterol. High blood sugar and high insulin levels cause the artery lining to produce greater amounts of a strong vasoconstrictor called endothelin-1; it causes the arteries to constrict leading to high blood pressure.

Sugar is sticky and excess sugar in the bloodstream attaches itself to proteins to form Advanced Glycosylation Endproducts (AGEs). AGEs bind to the inner lining of arteries and stimulate them to produce inflammatory chemicals; this causes damage to the artery walls which promotes the development of atherosclerosis. AGEs promote the formation of free radicals in the body. Diabetics also produce more of the chemicals that stimulate blood clots. Advanced atherosclerotic plaques in arteries are more likely to rupture and lead to a clot and complete blockage of an artery in diabetics.

If you are a diabetic you need to be following a low carbohydrate, high protein eating plan. The plan in the book *"Can't Lose Weight? Unlock The Secrets That Keep You Fat"* will help you to achieve better blood sugar control, lose weight and reverse a fatty liver. For best results, you should follow this eating plan under the guidance of a qualified naturopath or nutritionist. For more information on eating plans please call our Health Advisory on 623 334 3232.

• Cigarettes and Other Toxins

Cigarettes contain thousands of toxic chemicals, many of which are able to cause direct damage to the lining of our arteries, through their irritant action. This makes the arteries much more likely to accumulate fatty deposits, calcium and other debris.

We also generate a great deal of toxins within our own body. A toxic colon will create a toxin filled body. If we have too much bad bacteria and not enough good bacteria in our intestines (a condition called dysbiosis), these bad bugs can produce an endotoxin called lipopolysaccharide; it is one of the most inflammatory substances in the body. Our body uses HDL "good" cholesterol to bind to and neutralize endotoxins (toxins generated within our body), therefore having a lot of toxins in our body will use up HDL and leave us with low levels of this protective cholesterol.

We are also exposed to a great deal of toxins in our environment, such as plastic, pollution, heavy metals and pesticides. If our liver does not detoxify these substances well enough we will be left with a very toxic bloodstream and tissues. These toxins all generate free radicals in our body, use up valuable antioxidants and promote systemic inflammation. If you feel you are suffering with toxin overload you are best off to follow the two week deep cleansing detox diet in our book *"The Ultimate Detox".*

• Stress

When we are stressed, our adrenal glands release the hormone adrenaline. This hormone promotes the production of the inflammatory chemicals interleukin-6 and interleukin-10. It also uses up vitamins B6, B12 and folic acid in our body, thus makes it more likely for homocysteine levels to rise. High homocysteine levels irritate our artery walls and promote atherosclerosis.

When we are stressed our adrenal glands also release the hormone cortisol. When the stress passes, cortisol levels go back down again. However, many of us live with chronic stress, and this means our cortisol levels remain chronically elevated. Cortisol interferes with the action of insulin, and in time can make us develop Syndrome X and high blood pressure. Cortisol in excess tends to make us gain weight in the abdominal area; excess weight in this region is a major risk factor for diabetes and heart disease.

When stress is present long term, it often leads to depression. It is thought that cortisol is the link between depression and heart disease. A recent study done on over 2 800 men and women over age 55 showed that minor depression increases the risk of a heart attack by 60 percent, and major depression triples the risk of a fatal heart attack. Ref.74. Stress generates a lot of free radicals in our body and makes us use up vitamins and minerals at a much faster rate.

• Infections

An infection will raise the amount of inflammation in your body because of the toxins that bacteria and viruses produce, and because of the chemicals our immune cells produce in response to an infection. People suffering with an infection usually have higher levels of C-reactive protein (CRP) in their body, which is a major risk factor for heart disease. A study published in the *New England Journal of Medicine* analyzed 40 000 medical records and found that some respiratory tract infections and urinary tract infections can trigger a heart attack or stroke. Cystitis and pneumonia were the infections studied, and it was found that in susceptible people the chance of having a heart attack or stroke was much higher in the three days after having a respiratory tract infection.

If you have an elevated level of CRP and you don't know why, it is quite possible you have a hidden infection in your body. Bacteria, viruses and other infectious agents can produce toxins that cause irritation and injury to the walls of your arteries. This sets the stage for the development of atherosclerosis. Various imaging techniques have allowed doctors to detect microorganisms in the fatty plaques of arteries. Bacterial toxins, cytokines and other chemicals secreted by white blood cells during infections are detected in high amounts in many patients who have recently had a heart attack or stroke.

The bugs suspected of being able to promote heart disease include Helicobacter pylori, the bacterium linked to stomach ulcers; Chlamydia pneumoniae, which can cause pneumonia and bronchitis; Herpes Simplex type 1, the virus that causes cold sores; various bacteria that can cause gum disease; and cytomegalovirus, a very common viral infection that usually produces no symptoms at all.
It is very important to have a strong functioning immune system, as this will help to protect you against infections. It is often chronic, long standing infections that do the most harm.

• **Immune Dysfunction**
Allergies and autoimmune diseases leave our immune system in a hyper-stimulated state. Redness, swelling, discharge, itching and pain are all typical symptoms of these conditions, and they indicate that there is a lot of inflammation in your body. It is important to work on strengthening your immune system, as chronic inflammation like this wrecks havoc on your body, and generates an enormous amount of free radicals. Your body is in a constant state of stress if it is always battling with allergies or an autoimmune condition. The chemicals released into the bloodstream of people who suffer with allergies or autoimmune diseases include cytokines, prostaglandins, leukotrienes and thromboxanes. These

substances promote inflammation of the artery walls, and make blood clots much more likely.

If you suffer with an allergy such as eczema, hayfever, sinusitis, or an autoimmune disease such as rheumatoid arthritis, Hashimoto's thyroiditis or lupus, you may be much more susceptible to heart disease than people who don't suffer from one of these conditions.   Various studies have shown that people with lupus and rheumatoid arthritis are at much greater risk of heart disease. People with Systemic Lupus Erythematosis (SLE) are between 7 and 50 times more likely to have a heart attack than the general population. Ref.75, 76. This increased risk is independent of traditional risk factors such as high cholesterol and smoking.

• High Blood Pressure
This is a well known classic risk factor for heart disease and stroke because it places greater stress on your arteries, and in time weakens them. However, we now know that hypertension promotes inflammation in the body. Angiotensin 2 is a type of protein made in the body that raises blood pressure by causing constriction of the blood vessels, as well as sodium retention by the kidneys. Many common blood pressure medications work by inhibiting angiotensin converting enzyme, the enzyme responsible for producing angiotensin 2. It has recently been discovered that angiotensin 2 is also capable of causing inflammation to the inner lining of our arteries (endothelium). It promotes the production of free radicals by the cells that line our arteries, and also makes these cells release sticky molecules that make it more likely for LDL cholesterol and other substances to bind to them. Ref.77

We also know that if you have high blood levels of C-reactive protein, you are more likely to develop high blood pressure because CRP reduces nitric oxide production by the endothelial cells, (cells lining the artery walls). Nitric oxide dilates our blood vessels and reduces inflammation inside them.

Is Aspirin the Answer?

Aspirin is a non-steroidal anti-inflammatory drug. It is in a class of drugs called salicylates, and works by inhibiting the release of chemicals in the body that cause pain and inflammation. In addition to its use for acute conditions such as headache, fever or period pain, small doses of aspirin are often used to prevent heart attacks and strokes in high risk individuals. Aspirin has a blood thinning effect, and in this way may reduce the chance of a blood clot blocking a blood vessel and causing a heart attack or stroke. For this purpose aspirin is taken in a smaller dose, usually 80-100mg. Popular brands include Bayer Low Dose Aspirin, Ecotrin and St. Joseph.

However, aspirin is not without potential side effects, and there are questions as to whether it really reduces the risk of heart attack and stroke at all. Possible side effects of aspirin include upset stomach, abdominal cramps, skin rash, allergic skin reactions, and it contributes to the development of leaky gut syndrome; making food allergies more likely to develop. A potential serious side effect of aspirin is gastrointestinal bleeding. According to Dr John Reckless, chairman of Heart UK, "If you put the average older patient on aspirin in one year, one person in 262 would have a significant gastrointestinal bleed in that one year". One possible symptom of gastrointestinal bleeding is black or bloody stools. If you experience this symptom it is vital you see your doctor as soon as possible.

The Women's Health Study, which ran for ten years found that regular use of low dose aspirin does not prevent first heart attacks in women younger than 65. The group of women who took 100 milligrams of aspirin every other day were no less likely to have a heart attack than the group taking a placebo. Each group had approximately 20, 000 participants. Most previous studies showing aspirin to reduce the risk of heart attacks and strokes were done on men. The women in the study who took aspirin had a forty percent greater chance of suffering severe gastrointestinal bleeding, and they also experienced more minor bleeding and bruising. Interestingly, the incidence of hemorrhagic stroke was greater in the women who took aspirin. This is the type of stroke caused by bleeding, not blockage due to a blood clot. This makes sense since aspirin reduces the ability of the blood to clot. Therefore, if you are a woman without significant risk of heart disease, it is not recommended you take aspirin as a preventative. Ref.78

An interesting study called "The warfarin/aspirin study in heart failure" was published in the *American Heart Journal*. Patients with congestive heart failure are considered to be at increased risk of suffering a heart attack or stroke. This particular study involved 279 patients who were diagnosed with heart failure that required medication with diuretics. The patients were divided into three groups, aspirin therapy, warfarin therapy, and no blood thinning therapy. The results of the study showed no health benefits from aspirin or warfarin to these patients; there was no difference in deaths, or non-fatal heart attacks or strokes. Significantly more patients taking aspirin were hospitalized because of worsening heart failure. The conclusion of this study was *"Antithrombotic therapy in patients with heart failure is not evidence based but commonly contributes to polypharmacy"*. This means that there are no proven benefits to taking blood thinning medications in patients with heart failure, and they increase the risk of side effects from adverse drug interactions. Ref.79

A daily aspirin may reduce the risk of heart attacks and strokes in some individuals. However there are much safer and healthier ways to thin your blood. The omega 3 fats found in fish oil, flaxseed oil and walnuts have a powerful blood thinning effect. All antioxidants help to thin the blood; you can obtain these through regularly consuming raw vegetable juices and garlic, and taking supplements of vitamin E. Do not take vitamin E, garlic or ginkgo biloba supplements if you are on blood thinning medication without consulting your doctor.

Chapter Ten

THE TESTS YOU MUST HAVE TO DETERMINE YOUR RISK OF HEART DISEASE

Now that you know there are many other risk factors for heart disease than high cholesterol, you need to know which tests to ask your doctor for. The following are tests you should request if you have heart disease, or are concerned about developing it:

Blood Lipids/Fats

TYPE OF CHOLESTEROL	NORMAL REFERENCE RANGE
Total cholesterol	<200mg/dL Desirable
	200-239mg/dL Borderline High
	≥240mg/dL High
HDL cholesterol	38-72mg/dL (Male)
	46-87mg/dL (Female)
LDL cholesterol	<100mg/dL Optimal
	100-129mg/dL Near Optimal
	130-159mg/dL Borderline High
	160-189mg/dL High
	≥190mg/dL Very High
Total cholesterol/HDL ratio	Below average: 2.5-3.6
	Average: 3.7-5.5
	High: 5.6-8.3
	Very high: >8.3
Triglycerides	9-177mg/dL
Lipoprotein (a)	less than 30mg/dL

A blood test for cholesterol must include the different fractions; a total cholesterol only figure is quite meaningless. An ideal total cholesterol level is around 183-214mg/dL, any lower than 179mg/dL is not desirable. Your HDL cholesterol should be as high as possible, and your LDL cholesterol should be as low as possible. It is normal to have more LDL than HDL in our body though.

Another important measure is the total cholesterol to HDL ratio. You want this figure to be as low as possible. This ratio is determined by dividing your total cholesterol by your HDL. For example, if your total cholesterol is 191mg/dL and your HDL cholesterol is 62mg/dL, 191 divided by 62 = 3.1. This means your total cholesterol/HDL ratio is 3.1, indicating you have a low risk of heart disease.

Your triglycerides should be as low as possible. High blood levels of triglycerides make your bloodstream thick and sticky, and make clots much more likely to occur.

Lipoprotein (a) is a molecule of LDL cholesterol bound to a protein called apolipoprotein (a). It is a major risk factor for heart disease; much more significant than other blood fats. People with high levels usually get atherosclerosis early in life. Ref.80.

A blood lipid test should always be done in a fasting state, where you have not eaten for 12 hours prior to the test.

In Canada cholesterol and triglycerides are tested in a different unit of measurement; they are tested in millimoles per liter.
To convert mg/dL of HDL or LDL cholesterol to mmol/L, divide by 39.

To convert mg/dL of triglycerides to mmol/L, divide by 89.

Heart Association Recommendations for At Risk Individuals

The American Heart Association has a different set of reference ranges for several tests, for what are called "at risk individuals". The criteria you must meet to be an "at risk individual" include:

- Known coronary artery disease

- Other known signs of atherosclerosis such as peripheral artery disease (eg. Intermittent claudication), blocked carotid arteries (which lead to the brain), or aortic aneurysms.

- Diabetes mellitus

- Chronic kidney failure, or kidney transplantation

- Familial hypercholesterolemia (a genetic disorder)

- Familial combined hyperlipidemia (another kind of genetic disorder)

- HDL <40mg/dL

- Significant family history of heart disease (CHD in male first degree relative <55 years; CHD in female first degree relative <65 years).

- High blood pressure (hypertension) ≥140/90mmHg or on blood pressure medication

- Overweight or obesity

- Cigarette Smoking

- Impaired fasting glucose (blood sugar level between 110 and 124mg/dL)

- Age (≥45 years for men; ≥55 years for women).

- Below normal levels of albumin in the blood and/or impaired kidney function.

The following table states the LDL "bad" cholesterol goal for higher risk individuals:

Risk factors	LDL cholesterol goal
Coronary heart disease or Diabetes.	<100mg/dL
2 or more other risk factors	<130mg/dL
0-1 risk factors	<160mg/dL

According to the American Heart Association, lowering LDL cholesterol is the most important factor in reducing the risk of coronary heart disease.

Blood Sugar and Insulin

Testing your blood sugar level is vital, as diabetes is a major risk factor for heart disease and ischemic stroke. Even if you are not classified as a diabetic, a higher than normal blood sugar level means you have poor glucose tolerance, or your body does not regulate your blood sugar well. This is a forerunner to diabetes.

Having elevated blood insulin levels may indicate that you have insulin resistance; also called Syndrome X or metabolic syndrome. This is much more likely if you are overweight, especially in your abdominal area. Having your insulin levels checked is a good preview, to see if you are likely to have blood sugar problems in the future.

These tests must be done in a fasting state.

Blood glucose level	65-109mg/dL normal	110-124mg/dL impaired glucose tolerance	Over 124mg/dL Diabetes
Blood insulin level	<10mU/L normal	>10mU/L = insulin resistance	

In Canada blood glucose is measured in millimoles per liter. To convert mg/dL of glucose to mmol/L, divide by 18 or multiply by 0.055.

C-Reactive Protein

This is the most important test you need, as it is the biggest risk factor for coronary heart disease. Even if your cholesterol and triglyceride levels are low or normal, and you don't have any of the traditional risk factors for heart disease, an elevated CRP level is cause for concern. Your level of CRP should be as low as possible. This is a test that your doctor will often miss.

Desirable level: 0.0-5.0mg/L

Homocysteine

This is another often overlooked test, but is essential to evaluate your true risk of heart disease. High levels of homocysteine in your bloodstream have an abrasive effect on your artery walls, making it more likely that fatty particles and other substances will cling to them. This initiates the development of atherosclerosis. You will have higher blood levels of homocysteine if you don't consume enough vitamins B6, B12 and folic acid. They are found in most fruits and vegetables as well as animal foods. Other possible causes of raised homocysteine are listed in chapter eight.

This test must be done in a fasting state.
Desirable range: 6.0-14.0 μmol/L

Thyroid Function Test

An underactive thyroid gland, called hypothyroidism is extremely common, and actually affects one third of post-menopausal women. If your thyroid gland is underactive, all metabolic processes in your body slow down. You will probably gain weight, and the metabolism of cholesterol slows down too. This means that your cholesterol level may rise, even if you don't have other risk factors for high cholesterol. Thankfully it is easy to treat thyroid problems safely and adequately. When this occurs, cholesterol levels usually normalize by themselves.

HORMONE	NORMAL REFERENCE RANGE
Thyroid stimulating hormone (TSH)	0.5-5.0mU/L
Free T 4	9.0-24.0pmol/L
Free T 3	2.2-5.4pmol/L

Blood pressure

If your blood pressure is too high, a great deal of stress is placed on your arteries, as blood whooshes through them at increased pressure. Eventually small tears occur in the inner lining (endothelium) of your arteries. This makes them stickier and it is more likely that fats and other substances in your bloodstream will cling to your arteries, starting atherosclerosis. Hypertension is a major risk factor for stroke as well as heart attacks.

The most common apparatus used to measure blood pressure is called a sphygmomanometer. An ideal blood pressure is considered 120/80 mmHg; referred to as 120 over 80. The top reading is the systolic value and indicates the pressure of blood in your arteries during a contraction of the left ventricle of the heart. The bottom reading is the diastolic value, and indicates the pressure inside your arteries when the heart is at rest.

Nearly one in three US adults have high blood pressure. Blood pressure is classified as "high-normal" if it is between 120/80 and 140/90 mmHg. You are considered to have high blood pressure if your reading is above 140/90 mmHg. It is best not to smoke or consume caffeine containing foods such as coffee for two hours before this test, as it may give a falsely high reading. Anxiety will have the same effect. It is normal for blood pressure to rise as we get older. If you have a strong family history of hypertension, it is very likely you will be affected also. It is essential to treat high blood pressure, as it is dangerous; medication is very effective at this. Cholesterol lowering drugs do not lower blood pressure; our heart saving tips in chapter twelve can help normalize your blood pressure.

Pulse rate

This is a simple test you can do yourself to determine how well your heart is functioning. It will tell you how many times your heart beats per minute. Find your pulse on a location such as your wrist or neck, ask someone to time you for one minute and count how many times you feel your pulse beat in that time. Generally the slower your pulse, the fitter you are and the stronger your heart. The exceptions are if you have heart disease or a pacemaker. It is important to check your pulse after you have rested for some time, or first thing in the morning. Ideally it should be below 60, and definitely not above 70.

Chapter Eleven

MYTHS AND FACTS ABOUT FOODS AND FOOD LABELS

Don't Be Fooled by Food Labels

The labels on a lot of foods in the supermarket are very deceiving, and help to maintain a lot of misconceptions the public have about what is a healthy food and what isn't. No matter what the advertising on the label states, you must always read the ingredients list at the back and look at the nutrition panel. This will give you a true representation of what is really in the food you are eating.

The ingredients list will tell you exactly what is in the food, arranged in order by weight from most to least. The nutrition information panel will give you specific details on the nutrient content of the food. This can be quite confusing because everything is measured in grams. Most people cannot relate to grams unless they are a nutritionist or cocaine dealer! It will be easier to remember that one teaspoon holds an average of five grams. Therefore, if a breakfast cereal contains 11 grams of sugars per 30 grams, you will know that there are more than two teaspoons of sugar in a 30 gram serve. A sugary breakfast cereal like this may be extremely low in fat, but eating it will still make you fat and raise your risk of diabetes and heart disease significantly.

There are several breakfast cereals available that claim to do your heart good. The cereals contain a picture of a heart on the box, with statements about lowering cholesterol and/or blood pressure. Don't be fooled by the advertising claims; most of these breakfast cereals are extremely high in sugar, and some contain hydrogenated vegetable oil and artificial additives. Look carefully to see how many times sugar appears in the ingredient list; particularly as high fructose corn syrup.

Keep in mind that the "Nutrition Facts" panel contains the amount of nutrients in the food per serving size. If you eat two or three times the recommended serving size (which isn't hard for many foods), you will need to double or triple the grams of carbohydrate, fat and protein you have eaten. The percentage of daily value figure on the label is based on a 2 000 calorie a day diet. Most people don't know how many calories they eat each day, and in fact many people eat a lot more than this.

Reading food labels

Below you will find some common statements on food labels and learn how they can be misleading:

Cholesterol free:
It is common to find this term on the packaging of many varied foods. Some examples include hot potato snacks like fries, wedges and hash browns; potato crisps and corn chips; margarine, vegetable oil and even avocados.

First of all cholesterol is produced in the cells of the liver, small intestine, and in tiny amounts by other cells. For this reason cholesterol is only found in animal foods; an avocado cannot possibly contain cholesterol since it doesn't have a liver! Many of the foods labeled cholesterol free are actually cooked in refined vegetable oil such as canola oil, sunflower, soybean or safflower oil. The oils used are processed in a way that damages their fatty acid content, produces trans fatty acids and leaves them rancid (oxidized). These fats are highly unstable and act as free radicals in your body; they damage your cell membranes, DNA and inner lining of your blood vessels. So even if the oven fries are baked and not fried, are cooked in polyunsaturated vegetable oil, and have a Heart Association tick on the pack, they are doing your heart a great deal of damage. Potatoes are very high in carbohydrate also, and increase your risk of heart disease by promoting Syndrome X.

All margarines are cholesterol free, yet they are still bad for your heart because they are made of refined, rancid vegetable oil and many contain trans fatty acids. It doesn't matter which vegetable oil the margarine is made of; whether it is olive oil, canola oil or soy oil, it is the processing of this oil and the hardening (hydrogenation) which damages the fats and makes them unhealthy. You are much better off using cold pressed extra virgin olive oil or butter, rather than margarine. Don't think you are getting any of the benefits of soy by using a margarine made from its oil; soy oil does not contain any phyto-estrogens, and both it and canola oil are typically genetically engineered. Remember that the cholesterol in your diet has very little effect on your blood levels of cholesterol, and you do not need to eat any cholesterol to have high blood levels of this substance.

Low fat:
There are a huge amount of low fat foods filling the supermarket shelves, ranging from yogurt, to packet soup to breakfast bars. The problem with low fat foods is that they are nearly always higher in carbohydrate than their regular counterparts. Once the fat is gone, sugar or starch is usually added in its place to improve the texture and mouth-feel of the product.

Low fat foods are not very good at satisfying the appetite; you will probably be feeling hungry or craving something sweet fairly soon afterwards. High carbohydrate foods promote high blood insulin levels, which can lead to weight gain and the development of Syndrome X. You are better off eating the full fat variety of most foods.

High fructose corn syrup (HFCS) is a common addition to very many processed foods, especially low fat foods. Have a close look at food labels and you will be surprised how often this term appears. Fructose is the type of sugar present in fruit, but HFCS is artificially manufactured from corn starch and is used as a sweetener because it is cheaper than table sugar and tastes even sweeter. It has been used in American food since the 1970s and many researchers believe it is the cause of the obesity epidemic in the US.

The problem with HFCS is that fructose is converted into fat very quickly in the liver, and it raises both cholesterol and triglycerides. Studies done on rats have shown that the livers of rats consuming HFCS looked like the livers of alcoholics; they were clogged with fat and over time developed cirrhosis. In 2001 Americans consumed an average of 63 pounds of high fructose corn syrup each. Make sure you avoid foods containing this sweetener.

Suitable for frying, baking and roasting:
This expression is often found on a bottle of vegetable oil. The same oil will usually claim to be cholesterol free and/or free of saturated fat. Health authorities slam saturated fat as the main cause of high cholesterol levels, therefore if an oil is monounsaturated or polyunsaturated it must be healthy. This is false, as saturated fats are also formed in our body out of sugar we have eaten; you don't need to eat any fat at all to have high blood levels of saturated fat.

Do not use any vegetable oil unless it states it has been cold pressed and unrefined; extra virgin olive oil is your best choice. All other vegetable oils have been processed in a way that exposed them to oxygen, light and heat. Fatty acids are very delicate and susceptible to damage, and such processing turns the fat rancid, meaning it will create a lot of inflammation in your body. When these vegetable oils are heated, such as through frying, it causes significantly more damage to the oil. Have a look at the trans fatty acid content of vegetable oil in the nutrition panel; there is no safe level of trans fat intake.

Vegetable oil:
Many food labels will state the ingredient "vegetable oil" but not specify which vegetable oil is used. The answer is that cheap, highly refined oils like cottonseed, soy and corn oil are often used. Cottonseed oil is especially worrying; it is found widely in blended vegetable oils, baked foods, fried foods and snack foods. It is commonly used to cook donuts. As well as containing trans fats, cottonseed oil may be high in pesticide residues, as cotton is a heavily sprayed crop. Cottonseed oil is often contaminated with mycotoxins; these are fungal toxins that can cause cancer. If consumed in large quantities, this oil can be toxic to the liver and gallbladder. Ref.81

Foods you have been misled about

Eggs:
Eggs traditionally have a very bad reputation for promoting heart disease. Most people who are conscious of reducing their cholesterol either avoid eggs altogether, or limit their consumption to once a week. It is a myth that eating eggs will raise your cholesterol level. It is true that eggs contain cholesterol (approximately 215mg per egg) and saturated fat. However, most cholesterol in your body was made in your liver, and the cholesterol you consume in your diet has very little effect on your blood cholesterol level. A recent study published in the *American Journal of Clinical Nutrition* showed that significantly reducing your dietary

cholesterol consumption will only lower serum cholesterol levels by an average of one percent! Ref.82. That's definitely not worth the hard work!

Many studies have shown that egg consumption is not related to risk of coronary heart disease or stroke in men or women. Both the Framingham and Tecumseh long term studies have shown that those people who ate the most cholesterol had roughly the same blood cholesterol level of those who ate the least. Prominent heart researcher Ancel Keys had the following to say about dietary cholesterol: "There's no connection whatsoever between cholesterol in food and cholesterol in blood. And we've known that all along. Cholesterol in the diet doesn't matter at all unless you happen to be a chicken or a rabbit". Ancel Keys, Ph. D., professor emeritus at the University of Minnesota 1997. Ref.83

Eggs can become problematic if the cholesterol inside them gets oxidized. This can occur if eggs are cooked at high temperatures where the yolk is broken; examples of this include frying and omelets. The cholesterol in eggs should not become oxidized if you boil or poach them. Eggs are an excellent source of protein, and are a useful addition to a low carbohydrate diet. Eating eggs for breakfast will help to keep hunger at bay for hours, and will reduce cravings for sweets mid morning. Eggs are also high in the nutrient betaine, necessary to keep blood homocysteine levels low.

Coconut
Coconut has received a lot of negative press. Most of us consider it to be a fattening food, and one to avoid if we are trying to lose weight or lower our cholesterol. It is true that coconut contains a high amount of saturated fat; however, approximately half of this is lauric acid, which has been shown to not raise cholesterol levels. Lauric acid has antibacterial, antiviral and antiprotozoal properties, helping our immune system to overcome many types of infections. Chronic infections are a potent risk factor for heart disease, and coconut fat can help to strengthen our immune system. Traditional Asian cultures that rely heavily on coconut in their diet do not suffer with the diseases common in Western countries,

where low fat diets are encouraged.

A study published in 1981 examined the traditional diets of the people in two South Pacific Islands. The study began in the 1960s, when Western foods were not yet a part of the diet of either culture. Coconuts were a huge part of both diets; the saturated fat from coconut formed up to 60 percent of the calories consumed by these people. The study found that these populations were relatively healthy, and free of heart disease and obesity. The researchers found that "Vascular disease is uncommon in both populations, and there is no evidence of the high saturated fat intake having a harmful effect in these populations". Ref.84

A very interesting study titled "Choice of cooking oils – myths and realities" was done in India in response to the alarming rise in coronary heart disease and type 2 diabetes in this country. Indians have been encouraged to replace traditional saturated cooking fats like ghee and coconut fat with supposedly more "heart friendly" polyunsaturated oils like sunflower, safflower and corn oil. The research found that by increasing their intake of these omega 6 polyunsaturated vegetable oils, Indians are making themselves much more prone to the development of type 2 diabetes and heart disease. The study actually recommended that more traditional cooking fats be used in their place. Ref.85. Coconut is a very healthy addition to your diet; you can use coconut milk in cooking, or to make smoothies. Pure, unrefined coconut fat can be purchased from health food stores and used in place of vegetable oil when making stir fries and other Asian recipes.

Coffee

It's probably news you don't want to hear, but coffee is not the best thing for your heart. Coffee affects our metabolism in several ways that place us at increased risk of heart disease. One way that coffee increases our risk of heart disease is by promoting inflammation in our body. A study done in Greece recruited 1514 men (aged 18-87 years) and 1528 women (aged 18-89 years); their blood levels of inflammatory chemicals were analyzed in relation to coffee consumption. When compared to men who drank no coffee at all, men who consumed more than 200mL per day had a 50 percent higher level of interleukin-6 (IL6), a 30 percent higher C-reactive protein level, 12 percent greater serum amyloid-A, 28 percent higher tumor necrosis factor (TNF)-alpha levels and three percent higher white blood cell counts. For women who consumed 200mL per day of coffee, these figures were even higher. All of these chemicals are indicators of inflammation in the body, and are directly linked to higher rates of heart disease. Ref.86

Coffee also has the ability to raise blood pressure and damage our blood vessels. An Australian study was conducted on 18 healthy middle aged men and women who consumed 250mg of caffeine per day; this is roughly the amount found in two or three cups of coffee. The study showed that caffeine caused raised blood pressure and made the aorta less elastic and more rigid. Ref.87 The aorta is the largest artery in the body. People who drink coffee have higher amounts of the stress hormones cortisol and ACTH in their bloodstream than people who don't. Ref.88. These stress hormones can act as free radicals in our body and promote abdominal obesity.

Drinking unfiltered, boiled coffee can raise total cholesterol, LDL "bad" cholesterol and triglycerides if six or more cups are consumed per day. Ref.89 This effect is not present in filtered coffee, as it is the coffee oils found only in unfiltered or boiled coffee that are the culprit. Unfiltered coffee is more common in Europe; ground coffee is placed in a device that goes on the stovetop. Greek coffee is a type of unfiltered, boiled coffee. A more worrying fact is that coffee can raise homocysteine levels; four or more cups per day are required to have this effect. High homocysteine levels are a major risk factor for heart disease because homocysteine causes damage to artery walls and makes platelets stickier. Caffeine also promotes insulin resistance, meaning it makes us more likely to gain weight and develop diabetes. It is okay to enjoy coffee in moderation, approximately two to four cups a day.

Canola oil
Canola was originally developed from the rape seed. It was modified by selective breeding because rapeseed oil was too high in a toxic

fatty acid called erucic acid. Canadian plant breeders came up with a variety of rapeseed that is much lower in erucic acid, yet high in beneficial monounsaturated fat and omega 3 fat. Only olive oil contains more monounsaturated fat than canola oil. Canola oil also contains approximately ten percent of the omega 3 fat alpha-linolenic acid. The new modified canola oil was originally called LEAR oil; this stands for Low Erucic Acid Rapeseed. Both "LEAR" and "rape" don't have pleasant connotations, so a cleaver marketing guru came up with the name canola in 1978, alluding to Canadian oil.

Canola oil is now widely available as a cooking oil, in margarines, and is present in a great number of processed foods. Olive oil is a much healthier choice, but it is too expensive for the food industry to use in processed foods. Also, the fact that olive oil goes cloudy in cold temperatures makes it unappealing to the eye when used in some foods.

The majority of canola oil on the market is heavily processed. It goes through a process of refining, bleaching and degumming. This exposes the oil to oxygen, light, high temperatures and chemical solvents. Canola oil is fairly high in omega 3 fats, and these are most sensitive to processing, and likely to become damaged and form trans fatty acids. Therefore, canola oil can be higher in trans fats than other liquid vegetable oils. You are better off getting omega 3 fats from whole foods like fish, walnuts, flaxseeds and pumpkin seeds; all of which are also rich in antioxidants. Another problem with canola oil is that a great deal of it is genetically modified. There are several new varieties, such as Roundup Ready Canola, which is more tolerant to some herbicides and insecticides. Genetically modified canola has been approved for use in the United States. If you do use vegetable oil in cooking, it is best to stick to extra virgin olive oil or virgin coconut fat.

What about cholesterol lowering margarine?

The variety of margarines available in the supermarket has expanded enormously in recent times. Some margarine spreads have got added plant sterols or stanols and claim to be able to lower cholesterol absorption. Plant sterols are also known as phyto-sterols, and they include beta-sitosterol, campesterol and stigmasterol, among others. It is true that plant sterols can inhibit cholesterol absorption in our digestive tract (cholesterol is also a type of sterol), and in this way reduce cholesterol levels. Therefore, if you eat some cholesterol containing food, such as eggs at the same time as the margarine, you will absorb less cholesterol from the eggs than usual. Bile that is secreted into our small intestine in response to a meal contains a great deal of cholesterol. Some of this is excreted in bowel movements but a lot of it gets re-absorbed back into our bloodstream through the intestinal wall. The sterols in margarine prevent some of this re-absorption of cholesterol.

Plant sterols or stanols are a controversial topic. They are estrogen-like compounds found naturally in many plants, but they are also a waste product of pulp and paper mills. Research has shown that rivers downstream of wood-pulp factories can become contaminated with plant sterols and this affects the fertility of fish. Some fish became hermaphrodites and others switched gender! Ref.90, 91 Experiments in test tubes have shown these sterols to stimulate breast cancer cells. Ref.92 Back in the 60s these compounds were used to manufacture human sex hormones. Ref.93 Since plant sterols clearly have hormonal effects, possibly it isn't a good idea for every man, woman and child to be consuming them.

Some studies have shown that consumption of phyto-sterols reduces blood levels of vitamin E and beta-carotene. One study published in the *American Journal of Clinical Nutrition* found that plant sterols reduced the bioavailability of beta-carotene by 50 percent, and alpha-tocopherol (vitamin E) by 20 percent. Ref.94. What is the point of lowering your cholesterol if that is going to make you deficient in important antioxidants that have been shown to reduce your risk of heart disease and cancer?

Cholesterol lowering margarines are expensive; expect to pay more than five dollars a tub. To get the full benefits from them you would have to eat 25g a day, roughly a heaped tablespoon. Some spreads contain canola oil and some contain olive oil and are promoted to be healthier, as they contain monounsaturated fat. However you don't get as much olive or canola oil as you may think. Most canola spreads contain between 30 and 35 percent canola oil, and olive oil spreads typically contain only 22 to 23 percent olive oil. The rest of the product is made up of a vegetable oil blend; typically soybean oil, cottonseed oil, corn oil or palm oil. Low fat margarine spreads contain more water, and some even contain gelatin.

The vast majority of margarines have been made from refined vegetable oils that have been processed using heat and chemical solvents. This means they contain rancid fats and often some trans fatty acids. New manufacturing techniques have been able to get the trans fat content of margarine very low, and some margarines are free of trans fats altogether. However, there are much healthier, more natural options. It is possible to obtain plant sterols from more natural sources such as raw nuts and seeds, legumes and extra virgin olive oil. When combined with an appropriate liver friendly, low carbohydrate eating plan it is possible for most people to achieve a healthy cholesterol level.

Healthy alternative spreads
Remember that most bread is fairly high in carbohydrate, and eating too much of it can raise your cholesterol and triglycerides, as well as promote weight gain and Syndrome X. Eat bread in small quantities, and choose one that is made from stone ground flour and has a low glycemic index. The following are all suitable spreads to use:

- Fresh avocado
- Tahini
- Hummus
- Natural nut butter/paste such as peanut, almond, cashew, macadamia

or Brazil nut butter.

- Tomato paste
- Baba ganoush
- Extra virgin olive oil

Cholesterol reducing chews

You are now able to purchase sweet, fudge-like candy specifically designed to reduce your cholesterol. Each chew contains 0.85 grams of plant stanol esters, which inhibit cholesterol absorption in the intestines, just like cholesterol lowering spreads do. According to the label, you are best to eat between two and four chews per day, depending on how much cholesterol lowering spread you use. The goal is to consume 3.4 grams of plant stanol esters per day, as recommended by the National Cholesterol Education Program (NCEP).

These chews contain almost no fat; they are mostly composed of sugar, the first two ingredients being "sugar" and "corn syrup". The FDA has approved the following health claim: "Products containing 0.7 grams or more of plant stanol esters per serving, eaten two to three times per day with meals, may reduce the risk of heart disease as part of a diet low in saturated fat and cholesterol". It is a pity that people are afraid to eat natural foods that are high in plant stanols like nuts, seeds and olive oil, for fear of gaining weight. Instead they are willing to pay a high price for a sugar filled, artificially flavored processed food. People are generally not aware that sugar and carbohydrate in the diet are converted into saturated fat in our body anyway.

Olestra

Olestra is a fat-based fat substitute that was approved for use in certain snack foods by the FDA in January 1996. It is made by Procter & Gamble Co. and is marketed under the brand name *Olean*. Olestra contains no calories, yet behaves and tastes like fat. Regular fat is made of one molecule of glycerol attached to three molecules of fatty acids. In Olestra, the glycerol molecule has been replaced with sucrose, and there are six, seven or eight fatty acids attached to it. The fatty acids are derived from corn, soybean, cottonseed, palm or coconut oil. Because there are so many fatty acids attached to the central molecule (sucrose), digestive enzymes cannot break the molecule down in the time it takes to pass through the digestive tract.

Snack foods commonly cooked in Olestra include potato chips, tortilla chips, crackers, pretzels, microwave popcorn and other savory snacks; they will be labeled as light versions. The problem with Olestra is that it can cause loose stools, fecal incontinence and abdominal cramps in most people, depending on how much is consumed. It also inhibits the absorption of the fat soluble vitamins A, E, D, K as well as beta carotene, lycopene and other carotenoids. Carotenoids are found in brightly colored vegetables such as tomatoes, carrots and pumpkin, and are known to have cancer protective properties. Food manufacturers who choose to use Olestra must add vitamins A, E, D and K to the product, to compensate for this loss. Carotenoids are not required to be replaced. Originally, the FDA required all foods containing Olestra to display the following warning: "This product contains Olestra. Olestra may cause abdominal cramping and loose stools. Olestra inhibits the absorption of some vitamins and other nutrients. Vitamins A, D, E and K have been added".

However, in 2003 the FDA dropped the requirement for this warning statement on labels. Foods containing Olestra no longer need to contain this warning. It was thought that since fat soluble vitamins are added to these products, the warning statement is no longer warranted. However, the loss of carotenoids is not compensated for. According to Dr Walter Willett, nutritionist at the Harvard School of Public Health in Boston, consumption of Olestra containing foods may be linked to an increased risk of cancer, stroke and heart disease. According to Dr Willett, daily consumption of a one ounce serving of Olestra can lower blood carotenoid levels by as much as 50 to 70%. Low blood levels of carotenoids are associated with an increased risk of cardiovascular disease, cancers of the prostate, lung and uterus, as well as degenerative eye diseases that can lead to blindness, such as cataracts and macular degeneration. Ref. 95

Chapter Twelve

10 HEART SAVING TIPS YOU MUST FOLLOW

If you are really serious about getting your cholesterol down and avoiding heart disease, you must practice the recommendations below. These tips will either reduce inflammation in your body, or work directly on lowering your cholesterol level, thus helping to protect you from heart disease and stroke. Remember that it is inflammation which initiates damage to your artery walls in the first place. If this inflammation continues, and you do not consume enough antioxidants in your diet, various harmful substances in your bloodstream can become stuck to the inner lining of your arteries. Cholesterol is thought to have a protective role; it adheres to your damaged blood vessels as a way of patching up the damage. If you have a lot of the wrong kind of cholesterol in your bloodstream, as well as other harmful, oxidized fats, the plaque will grow until eventually it prevents blood from flowing freely through your arteries. The plaque can rupture, a blood clot can form and you suffer a heart attack or stroke.

These are the essential guidelines to follow to save your heart:

1. Eat Less Carbohydrate

This is probably the most important thing you can do to reduce your risk of developing heart disease. Consuming too much carbohydrate can lead to Syndrome X, which promotes weight gain and can lead to type 2 diabetes. Diabetics have much higher rates of heart disease than the general population.

The sad fact is that when most people want to lower their cholesterol level, they think they must follow a low fat diet. The problem with this is, when you reduce the fat you are eating, you have to compensate for that by eating more of something else; and that something is usually carbohydrate.

Carbohydrate rich foods are the staple of many people's diets. Bread, pasta, rice, cereals, potatoes, corn, and all foods containing grains are high in carbohydrate; sugar is the most concentrated form of carbohydrate. All of these carbohydrate foods are digested into sugar in our body. In order for the sugar to enter our cells and be used for energy, our pancreas must release the hormone insulin. Over time the cells of our body can become resistant to the action of insulin, therefore the carbohydrate we eat is turned into fat. Insulin therefore is a fat creating hormone, and in this way a low fat, high carbohydrate diet can give us cravings and make us gain weight. The liver converts excess carbohydrate we consume into triglycerides and "bad" LDL cholesterol.

Numerous studies have shown that low fat diets can raise our triglycerides. The American Heart Association states that "Triglyceride levels consistently increase in response to short-term consumption of a very low fat diet". By "very low fat diet" they mean keeping fat intake to 15% of calories, protein to 15% of calories and carbohydrate to 70%. The American Heart Association goes on to say that the increase in triglycerides due to a very low fat diet is variable, but typically is 70%, and that high triglycerides are often accompanied by low levels of "good" HDL cholesterol. So there you have it, low fat diets are bad for your blood fats.

On the other hand, following a low carbohydrate diet can help you to lose weight, as well as get your blood cholesterol and triglyceride levels down; numerous studies have shown this. If you base your diet on salads and vegetables, lean meat, fish, chicken, eggs, along with small amounts of raw nuts and seeds, legumes and good fats such as olive oil, you should be able to lower your cholesterol and triglyceride levels. You can find an easy to follow low carbohydrate eating plan in the book called *"Can't Lose Weight? Unlock The Secrets That Keep You Fat"*.

A study published in the *Annuals of Internal Medicine* compared the effect on weight loss and hyperlipidemia (elevated blood fats) of a low carbohydrate ketogenic diet and a low fat diet. A ketogenic diet is where carbohydrate intake is severely restricted to between 20 and 40 grams per day; this means the diet is mainly composed of lean meat, fish, chicken and eggs, with small amounts of salad vegetables. In this study participants on the low carbohydrate diet kept carbohydrate intake to less than 20 grams per day; the low fat group kept fat intake to below 30% of calories, (this equates to less than 67 grams of fat per day for the average person who consumes 2000 calories per day). The low fat diet group had to eat less than 300mg of cholesterol daily, and both groups participated in exercise.

The results showed that a greater number of people in the low carbohydrate group stuck with the diet than people in the low fat group (76% versus 57%). After 24 weeks, weight loss was greater in the low carbohydrate group than the low fat group (average weight loss of 12.9% versus 6.7% of body weight). The interesting point is that triglycerides came down by 33mg/dL in the low carbohydrate group, and only 12mg/dL in the low fat group, and HDL cholesterol increased by an average of 5.5mg/dL in the low carbohydrate group, and actually decreased by 1.6mg/dL in the low fat group.

In basic terms, triglycerides decreased more, and HDL increased more in the low carbohydrate group compared to the low fat group. Ref.96. The low carbohydrate diet used here was quite extreme; it is not necessary to lower carbohydrate intake so severely to obtain good results. Another study published in the *Journal of the American Medical Association* compared a low glycemic diet with a low fat diet. In the study 39 overweight or obese patients between the ages of 18 and 40 participated. Weight loss results were similar in this study; however participants in the low glycaemic group experienced less hunger, less insulin resistance, lower triglycerides, lower C-reactive protein and lower blood pressure than those on the low fat diet. Re.97. Clearly lowering the amount of carbohydrate you eat can help you to feel less hungry, lose weight and improve your blood fats. If you would like help following a low carbohydrate diet, please phone our Health Advisory Service on 623 334 3232

The effect carbohydrates have on liver function

Eating more carbohydrate than we need results in its storage as body fat. The liver is the main fat metabolizing organ in the body, and excess carbohydrates are converted into fat in the liver; you will remember that most cholesterol in our body is manufactured in the liver. Over time, a high carbohydrate diet clogs our liver with fat and we can develop what is known as fatty liver disease; also known as non-alcoholic steatohepatitis. This is an extremely common condition, and affects an average of 20 percent of the population. Most people do not develop a fatty liver because they eat too much fat, they get it from eating too much sugar, bread, pasta, cereals, soft drinks, and other foods high in sugar which their liver turns into fat. Hydrogenated vegetable oil, which contains trans fatty acids also contributes to the development of fatty liver.

When we develop a fatty liver, it often causes us to have raised liver enzymes; this indicates that there is inflammation occurring in our liver. C-reactive protein is manufactured in the liver in response to inflammation, and it promotes further inflammation in the rest of our body, including our artery walls. If you need specific treatment to address a fatty liver, you will find the book *"The Liver Cleansing Diet"* very helpful.

2. Eat More Fiber

This is the best way you can get rid of some of the cholesterol in your body. One of the most important functions of cholesterol in our body is bile production. Bile is composed of bile salts, phospholipids (lecithin) and cholesterol. We need bile because it helps us to digest fat by emulsifying it inside our intestines; bile breaks fat into smaller globules so that fat digesting enzymes can work on it. The majority of the cholesterol that enters our intestines in bile is reabsorbed back into the bloodstream and goes to the liver again; however some of it is lost in bowel motions.

If you suffer with constipation, and have small infrequent stools, you won't be excreting nearly as much cholesterol as someone who has regular full bowel movements. Drinking between eight and ten glasses of pure water each day is important for healthy bowel function, but so is fiber. Fiber is non-digestible carbohydrate that comes from plants and passes straight through our body. There are two main types of fiber: insoluble and soluble. Insoluble fiber absorbs water in our intestines and swells, thus gives us bulkier stools. Wheat and rye are high in insoluble fiber. Soluble fiber is broken down by bacteria in the large intestine, helping to feed and nourish them; it also gives us a softer, bulkier stool. Soluble fiber is found in oats, barley, legumes and most fruits and vegetables. Pectin is one type of soluble fiber especially good at binding to cholesterol and removing it from our body; it is found mainly in apples, citrus fruits and onions.

Fiber is also very good at reducing your chances of developing diabetes.

This is because fiber in your digestive tract slows down the absorption of sugar into your bloodstream. In this way it helps to lower the glycemic index of a meal and helps to keep you full for longer. This is why wholegrain bread has a lower glycemic index than white bread, and is more satiating. In this way high fiber foods help to keep your weight down, and keep your blood sugar level balanced.

How to incorporate more fiber into your diet

Beware of sugar filled breakfast cereals and other heavily processed foods that claim to be high in fiber. You are best off getting fiber from wholesome, unprocessed foods. Oats are a great source of fiber, and are known to be able to lower cholesterol levels. Psyllium is extremely high in fiber, and is very good at binding cholesterol in the intestines and taking it out of the body. If you have high cholesterol and/or suffer with Syndrome X it is best to limit your consumption of grains, as they are high in carbohydrate, which is digested into sugar.

Legumes are an excellent source of fiber, and they are higher in protein and lower in carbohydrate than grains. Good choices include kidney beans, chick peas and lentils. All nuts and seeds provide plenty of fiber; examples include pecans, almonds, Brazil nuts, sunflower seeds, as well as ground linseeds.

Among vegetables, cucumbers, tomatoes and broccoli provide the most fiber. Fruits richest in fiber include berries, passionfruit, pears and apples. Seaweed is another good source of fiber; as well as binding cholesterol, the fiber in seaweed can bind to toxins in your gut and take them out of your body. Nori, wakame and arame are the most common types of seaweed available; you should be able to find them in health food stores, or the health food, or Asian food isle of a supermarket.

3. Eat the right fats and avoid the bad ones

Obtain Omega 3 Fats in Your Diet

An enormous amount of research has been done on the benefits of omega 3 fats for cardiovascular health. Omega 3 fatty acids are a type of polyunsaturated fatty acid with strong anti-inflammatory properties. As well as benefiting the heart, omega 3 fats are particularly good for helping arthritis, cognitive function and depression.

Alpha-linolenic acid (ALA) is an essential fatty acid found in flaxseeds, walnuts and other seeds and vegetables. Our cells convert ALA into two omega 3 fatty acids called eicosapentaenoic acid (EPA) and docosahexaenoic acid (DHA); they are especially abundant in brain cells, the retina of the eyes, adrenal gland and sex glands (ovaries and testes). In addition to making them in our cells, we can obtain EPA and DHA by eating oily fish such as salmon, sardines, herrings, mackerel, tuna and halibut.

Omega 3 fatty acids have the following benefits for our heart:

- They make our platelets less sticky, therefore reducing the risk of blood clots forming which can lead to a heart attack or stroke.

- They lower blood triglyceride levels.

- They decrease the risk of cardiac arrhythmias (disturbances in the heart's rhythm that can lead to a heart attack).

- They lower blood pressure.

- They decrease the rate of plaque accumulation in the arteries.

- They help to stabilize arterial plaques, making them less likely to rupture and lead to a heart attack.

- They increase levels of HDL "good" cholesterol.

- They can help to break up blood clots already present. Ref.98

A study published in the *Journal of the American Medical Association* evaluated more than 84 000 women and found those who ate fish five or more times per week had a 34 percent lower chance of coronary heart disease than women who ate fish less than once a month. Ref.99. In another study, patients with high cholesterol were given either EPA and DHA or a placebo for seven weeks. The patients who took EPA and DHA were found to have a significant improvement in the elasticity of their arteries. This means their blood pressure was likely to be lower, and they had a lower chance of blockages in their arteries. Ref.100

How you can get more omega 3 fats into your diet

Oily fish such as sardines, salmon, herrings, mackerel, anchovies and tuna are great sources of EPA and DHA. Much of the fish in our oceans today is contaminated with high levels of heavy metals, such as mercury and cadmium, as well as pesticides and industrial chemicals. Therefore, it is wiser to choose fish that is smaller, and lower down in the food chain. Larger fish at the top of the food chain have accumulated a lot of toxins in their bodies from all the smaller fish they have eaten. The healthiest fish are actually sardines and anchovies because they feed on plankton. However, if you can't stomach certain species of fish, you will still get benefits from eating any type you do like.

There are plenty of vegetarian sources of omega 3 fats; the best ones are:

- Ground flaxseeds. You can add these to smoothies, yogurt or sprinkle them on your cereal or fruit.
- Flaxseed oil. This can be used as a salad dressing or added to smoothies. Make sure you never heat flaxseed oil, as it is very susceptible to oxidation.

- Walnuts.
- Green leafy vegetables.
- Tofu.

Your body will have to convert the alpha-linolenic acid (ALA) in these foods to EPA and DHA.

If you feel that you need more omega 3 fats than your diet provides, you can take a fish or flaxseed oil supplement. An ideal dose would be three grams per day; this usually equates to three capsules.

Saturated fats are not as bad as you think. It is quite okay to include small amounts of them in your diet. Saturated fats are found predominantly in animal foods such as butter, full fat dairy products and red meat. Saturated fats have the following benefits:

- They provide structure and integrity to our cell membranes. Phospholipids are the type of fats making up our cell membranes, and they are made of mostly saturated fatty acids.
- They increase the satiety of a meal, helping to keep us full so that we don't over eat or binge on sweets.
- They enhance the function of our immune system.
- They are usually found in foods with essential fat soluble vitamins, such as vitamins A and D.
- They enhance our body's ability to use essential fatty acids.
- Even if you do not eat any saturated fats, your body will make them out of carbohydrate you ate.
- They have been part of the human diet for many generations, at a time when heart disease was nowhere near as prevalent as it is now.

Monounsaturated fats help to keep your heart healthy. Olive oil is one of the richest sources of monounsaturated fatty acids. If you use vegetable oil in cooking, olive oil is a good choice because it withstands high temperatures well. Other great sources of monounsaturated fats are hazelnuts, macadamia nuts, almonds, Brazil nuts, cashews, avocado and sesame seeds. Try to include all of these in your diet regularly.

A high intake of monounsaturated fat in Mediterranean countries is thought to be a reason they have such low rates of heart disease. This type of fat helps to lower cholesterol levels, and may offer some protection against cancer. Foods high in monounsaturated fat are often a good source of vitamin E as well.

Polyunsaturated fats are divided into two categories: omega 3 and omega 6. Omega 3 fats are highly beneficial and have been discussed above. The problem is that most people have far too much omega 6 fat in their diet. Vegetable oils high in omega 6 fatty acids include corn oil, soybean oil, cottonseed oil, sunflower oil and safflower oil. These are a fairly new addition to the human diet because of modern oil refining practices. These types of vegetable oils should never be used for cooking, as they are easily damaged by heat which causes them to be oxidized and act as free radicals in the body.

It is best to obtain polyunsaturated fats from whole foods, rather than refined oils. Suitable choices are sunflower seeds, pumpkin seeds, walnuts and sesame seeds. Flaxseed oil is high in omega 3 polyunsaturated fat and may be used as a salad dressing, in smoothies, or other ways as long as it is not heated.

Avoid Trans Fats

This is the worst kind of fat. We are continually being told that to reduce our risk of heart disease we must reduce our fat consumption, especially saturated fat. In its place we are encouraged to consume vegetable oil and vegetable margarine.
Just because vegetable oil comes from vegetables and is cholesterol free does not mean it is healthy for our heart. The main problem with vegetable oil is how it is processed. Modern manufacturing techniques

process the oil in a way that exposes it to high temperatures, oxygen, light and chemical solvents. This damages the fragile essential fatty acids in the oil, and creates many toxic components, including trans fatty acids. When these same oils are used to manufacture margarine, even more toxic by-products are created, and because the oil has been hardened, more trans fatty acids are usually created.

The harmful effects of trans fatty acids include:

Lower HDL "good" cholesterol.

Raise LDL "bad" cholesterol.

Raise lipoprotein (a).

Inhibit insulin binding, promoting obesity, Syndrome X and diabetes.

Interfere with various enzymes, including delta-6-desaturase, needed for essential fatty acid metabolism.

Promote cancer.

Promote the development of fatty liver.

Promote inflammation in the body by stimulating the release of inflammatory cytokines.

How to avoid trans fatty acids in your diet

The easiest way to do this is to avoid foods that state the words "vegetable oil" on the label. You can assume that this term means highly processed, poor quality, refined vegetable oil. The term "hydrogenated vegetable oil" usually means that the product contains trans fatty acids.

Vegetable fat usually means fully or partially hydrogenated vegetable oil, and should be avoided also.

Another problem with the term "vegetable oil" is that you don't know which vegetable oil in particular has been used; it is often cottonseed oil that is used in vegetable oil blends (such as cooking oil and margarine), fried or baked foods and snack foods. Cottonseed oil is very unhealthy; you can read about it in chapter eleven.

If you eat takeaway fried foods, you are guaranteed to be consuming large amounts of rancid, oxidized fats rich in trans fatty acids. In many restaurants cheap vegetable oil and margarine are used. The word "butter" on the menu usually means margarine because it is cheaper and has a longer shelf life. Always ask about the type of fat that your food is being cooked in. Extra virgin olive oil, butter and unrefined coconut fat (not copha) are the healthiest options.

The nutrition panel of many foods now lists the trans fat content of the food. There is no safe level of trans fat intake; they should be entirely avoided. By January 2006 the level of trans fats in all foods must be stated on the label.

4. Increase the Antioxidants in Your Diet

This is an extremely important component of protecting yourself against heart disease. We have always known that people who eat lots of fruit and vegetables are healthier and live longer than those who don't; now scientific research is discovering the reasons why. You may remember that cholesterol itself is not much of a problem to your health, rather it is oxidized (damaged by free radicals) cholesterol that causes all the damage to your artery walls. If you don't get enough antioxidants in your diet, there will be a lot of free radicals in your body, causing harm to your cell membranes, DNA, artery walls, and the various fats in your bloodstream. Antioxidants help to counteract the damaging effects of free radicals in our body. Free radicals occur naturally in our body, but toxins in our environment greatly increase the amount of these damaging substances.

Antioxidants found in foods, vitamins and minerals

A large Harvard University study in the USA of men and women found that people who eat eight or more servings of vegetables and fruit per day have a 20 percent lower chance of suffering heart disease than those who eat less than three servings. This study showed that every little bit helps, because for every one serving of fruit or vegetables per day, the risk of heart disease dropped by four percent! Ref.101.

It is important to eat as wide a variety of fruits and vegetables as possible, as they each have their own unique benefits. Try to include as many different colored fruits and vegetables as possible; make sure you include some leafy vegetables, some stem vegetables and some root vegetables. Consuming one raw vegetable salad each day is essential; many vital nutrients are destroyed by cooking.

Consuming plenty of plant foods will lower your blood C-reactive protein level. People who are fit, not overweight and eat plenty of fruits and vegetables have lower blood levels of this substance.

The power of juicing

One easy way to include more fruit and vegetables in your diet is through raw vegetable juicing. You will need to use a juice extractor and consume the juice as soon after making it as possible, as valuable nutrients are lost quickly once the juice has been made. Store bought vegetable juices in glass bottles or cartons are not a substitute because they are not raw juices. Fruit juices should be avoided, as they are far too high in sugar. You should be predominantly juicing vegetables, with a little fruit thrown in to improve the taste. Juicing vegetables breaks down the fibrous components and makes the nutrients present much easier to digest and more available to the body. There is very little effort required by your body to obtain the goodness in the vegetables. Unfortunately, with all the chemicals and stress we are exposed to these days, an average intake of fruits and vegetables is not enough to protect us from disease; juicing is essential! Juices are rich in so many essential nutrients, including vitamin C, beta-carotene, folic acid, B vitamins, vitamin K, potassium and magnesium. There really is no excuse not to consume them regularly. For some delicious juice recipes for your heart please see chapter fourteen.

Blueberries fight cholesterol

Researchers have discovered that the compound pterostilbene, found in blueberries works as effectively for lowering LDL "bad" cholesterol as the cholesterol lowering drug ciprofibrate. Ciprofibrate is in the class of cholesterol lowering drugs called fibrates; it is effective for lowering cholesterol but causes muscle pain and nausea in some people. Pterostilbene stimulates a receptor protein in liver cells which is responsible for lowering cholesterol and other blood fats. Blueberries do not cause any side effects, are delicious, high in fiber and help to protect your heart. Ref.102

Sweet news for chocoholics

If it makes you happy it can't be all bad; this is definitely the case with chocolate. Cocoa butter, which is present in chocolate, contains the saturated fat stearic acid. Even though it is a saturated fat, stearic acid does not raise LDL cholesterol; in fact it is converted into oleic acid in the liver. Ref.103. Oleic acid is a heart healthy monounsaturated fat present in high amounts in olive oil. I bet you didn't know that eating chocolate is another way of getting the benefits of olive oil!
Chocolate is quite high in antioxidants; it contains approximately 300

natural compounds. One of the most potent groups of antioxidants found in chocolate are called phenols; these are also present in red wine. Phenols in cocoa can prevent LDL cholesterol from building up in arteries and causing plaques. They can also inhibit the oxidation of cholesterol for up to two hours after consumption. Ref.104 The moral of the story is unfortunately not to eat chocolate every two hours; high levels of sugar and vegetable oil in some chocolate are its downfall. The darker the chocolate the higher it is in antioxidants; the higher the percentage of cocoa solids the better. You are best off eating small amounts of good quality dark chocolate, composed of 70 to 85 percent cocoa solids.

Red wine to cheer your heart

Many studies have been done on the benefits of red wine for the heart. One of the antioxidants found in red wine is called resveratrol. It is a type of polyphenol and is present in grape skins. Resveratrol is a powerful antioxidant that helps to protect cholesterol from oxidation, thus preventing it from doing harm to your arteries.

The polyphenols in red wine are also able to inhibit the production of endothelin-1; a type of protein that causes blood vessels to constrict and can make them more sticky, thus allowing fat and other substances to adhere to them and initiate atherosclerosis. Red wine is made from the flesh and skins of grapes, whereas white wine is only made from the flesh. It is the skins that give red wine its vibrant color. An ideal consumption of red wine would be one glass with a meal for women, and two glasses with a meal for men most days. It is best to have three alcohol free days per week.

Go nuts

Raw nuts and seeds are some of the healthiest foods you can eat. Even though they are fairly high in fat, it is the good monounsaturated and polyunsaturated fats. Nuts and seeds are also an excellent source of fiber and minerals; they should form a regular part of your diet. Suitable nuts include almonds, Brazil nuts, hazelnuts, walnuts, pecans, cashews, pine nuts and pistachios. Seeds include sunflower seeds, pumpkin seeds and sesame seeds. Peanuts are actually a legume, like peas and beans, but nutritionally they have similar properties to tree nuts. Nuts and seeds should be consumed un-roasted and un-salted. The fatty acids they contain are easily damaged by the heat of roasting.

Several studies have shown that people who eat nuts every week have better health and suffer less heart disease than people who eat nuts less often. The Nurses Health study was conducted in Boston, USA and assessed more than 86 000 women aged 34-59 years who were free of heart disease. The study found that women who consumed at least 140 grams of nuts per week had a 35 percent lower risk of coronary heart disease than women who ate less than 30 grams per month. Ref.105. Nuts and seeds have the ability to lower LDL "bad" cholesterol because of the good fats they contain; walnuts are especially helpful because they contain omega 3 fats. Most nuts and seeds are also a good source of folic acid, vitamin E and potassium; all essential for a healthy heart.

The Polymeal: A Tastier Alternative to the Polypill

The "Polypill" was an idea proposed by British researchers Wald and Law in 2003. It was to be an all in one drug that combines six drugs that act to lower cholesterol, lower blood pressure, aspirin to act as an anti inflammatory, and folic acid to lower homocysteine levels. The researchers claimed that if everyone over the age of 55 took this pill daily, rates of cardiovascular disease could be reduced by more than 80 percent. Ref.106. The Polypill generated a lot of publicity, but it has not been proven to be safe or effective. The biggest problems with it are cost, side effects (especially if the individual already takes other medication), and the fact that one dose cannot possibly suit everyone.

More recently, researcher Oscar Franco and colleagues have come up with the concept of the "Polymeal". This is a combination of foods that they claim can reduce cardiovascular disease by more than 75 percent if consumed daily. The Polymeal is a much safer alternative with no side effects. The foods it comprises are almonds, dark chocolate, fish, wine, fruits, vegetables and garlic.

The benefits of the components of the Polymeal are as follows:

Ingredient	% Risk reduction for cardiovascular disease
Wine 5oz/day	32%
Garlic 0.1oz/day	25%
Fruit & vegetables 14oz/day	21%
Dark chocolate 3.5oz/day	21%
Fish 4oz four times a week	14%
Almonds 2.4oz/day	12.5%

These results were obtained from data from the Framingham heart study and the Framingham offspring study. Ref.107

 A modified version of the Polypill, containing four drugs (two blood pressure drugs, a statin and aspirin) is to be trialled on patients with cardiovascular or cerebrovascular disease in Australia this year. The study will be funded by the National Health and Medicine Research Council (NHMRC). Ref.108. It may prove effective for some, but it is a lot less expensive, safer and tastier to include the above heart protective foods in your diet regularly.

The power of Vitamin C

Vitamin C is essential for the formation of collagen and elastin, needed to make our arteries strong. It is also one of the most powerful antioxidants in our body, with the ability to regenerate other antioxidants such as vitamin E and carotene. If we are deficient in vitamin C our connective tissue becomes weaker, this can result in bleeding gums, easy bruising, weakened arteries, excessive free radical damage in the body, and the oxidation of cholesterol and other fats in the body.

Dr Matthias Rath and Dr Linus Pauling have proposed a theory that the main cause of coronary heart disease is vitamin C deficiency. If we are deficient in vitamin C, our body's production of lipoprotein (a) increases. Raised lipoprotein (a) is a major risk factor for heart disease. It is a very similar molecule to LDL cholesterol, but it has a sticky repair protein attached to it called apo (a). If our blood levels of vitamin C go down, lipoprotein (a) and other repair proteins such as fibrinogen and fibrin build up in the artery walls, thickening them and making them stronger. This can become a problem because as the arteries thicken, they become narrower and less blood is able to flow through them.

Taking extra vitamin C is able to lower lipoprotein (a), fibrinogen and fibrin levels in the blood, thus preventing the arteries from thickening, and preventing atherosclerosis from developing. Sugar interferes with the activity of vitamin C in the body; this is just one more reason why eating too much sugar will give you heart disease. Other factors that deplete our body of vitamin C include smoking, stress and exposure to environmental pollution. Vitamin C supplements can improve the ability of blood vessels to dilate in patients with atherosclerosis, angina, congestive heart failure, high cholesterol and high blood pressure. Ref.109

You can ensure that you get plenty of vitamin C in your diet by eating RAW food each day, such as a raw vegetable salad and making a raw vegetable juice for yourself each day. All fruits contain vitamin C, especially rich sources include kiwifruit, cherries and oranges. If you do have diagnosed elevated lipoprotein (a) levels, high cholesterol or high C-reactive protein levels, you will need to take a vitamin C supplement. Because most of us are exposed to stress and environmental pollution, a supplement is probably essential. The best vitamin C supplements have added bioflavonoids and other antioxidants in the formula.

Co enzyme Q 10

This is a compound produced naturally in our body that is involved in energy production. It is found in the mitochondria of our cells (energy factories) and is required for the formation of ATP; our cells' major energy source. Co enzyme Q 10 is a powerful antioxidant, boosts the immune system and increases energy levels. Our body manufactures Co enzyme Q 10 in the same pathway that it manufactures cholesterol. Therefore, the cholesterol lowering drugs called statins inhibit the production of Co Q 10 in our body. It is believed that many of the side effects of cholesterol lowering drugs are actually Co enzyme Q 10 deficiency symptoms. Deficiency of Co Q 10 is strongly associated with congestive heart failure. This occurs when the heart becomes weak and is not able to pump blood around the body efficiently.

If you are taking cholesterol lowering drugs it is essential for you to take a Co Enzyme Q 10 supplement to make up for the loss caused by these drugs. Other benefits of Co Q 10 include the inhibition of blood clot formation, improved outcomes after heart surgery, and its antioxidant abilities, preventing oxidation of cholesterol. One study showed that patients who took a Co Enzyme Q 10 supplement within three days of having a heart attack were much less likely to have another heart attack and chest pain than patients who did not take a supplement. Ref.110. Co Q 10 has the ability to significantly lower blood lipoprotein (a) levels; this is a sticky type of blood fat that is a major risk factor for heart attacks. Ref.111

Policosanol

This is a dietary supplement produced from alcohols from sugar cane. It appears to be effective at lowering total cholesterol and LDL "bad" cholesterol, as well as raising HDL "good" cholesterol. Most studies done on the effects of policosanol were carried out in Cuba. It is known that policosanol inhibits cholesterol synthesis in the liver. The recommended dose is 10 to 20 milligrams after dinner. Unfortunately this supplement is fairly expensive.

5. Herbs to help your heart

Tea

Tea is the most widely consumed beverage after water, and archeological evidence suggests it was consumed 500 000 years ago, originally in China and India. Tea refers to the plant Camelia sinensis, and there are three main varieties: black, green and oolong. The difference between these is the way they are processed. Green tea is made from unfermented leaves, and contains the greatest amount of antioxidants. The leaves of black tea have been fully fermented, and oolong tea leaves are fermented for a shorter period of time.

Green tea is very high in a type of antioxidant called catechins. The main catechins found in green tea are epicatechin (EC), epigallocatechin (EGC), epicatechin gallate (ECG), and epigallocatechin gallate (EGCG). The last one is considered the most powerful, and research has proven it to have strong disease fighting properties. Tea drinkers appear to have a lower death rate after a heart attack than non tea drinkers Ref.112. Green tea was found to prevent the development of atherosclerosis in mice. Ref.113. This could be due to the antioxidants in it preventing the oxidation of cholesterol, and damage to the artery walls, and/or because tea has a dilating effect on the arteries.

A study published in the *Journal of Agriculture and Food Chemistry* analyzed the antioxidant activity of 22 vegetables as well as green and black tea. The researchers found that both green and black tea had much higher antioxidant activity against free radicals than all of the vegetables studied. Of the vegetables studied, garlic was the most powerful antioxidant, followed by kale, spinach, Brussels sprouts and broccoli. Ref.114

Eat your herbs and spices

A number of herbs and spices that are used in cooking actually have very powerful protective effects against heart disease.

Garlic has been used as a food and medicine in many cultures for thousands of years. First of all garlic is a strong antibiotic, it is able to kill a variety of bacteria, viruses, fungi and intestinal parasites. This is useful, as several infections have been associated with a higher risk of heart disease. If you eat garlic regularly, you are not likely to have hidden chronic infections in your body. Garlic is also a strong antioxidant, helping to protect our cells and tissues from damage and inflammation.

Studies have shown that garlic can help to prevent blood clots; it thins the blood, helps to lower cholesterol and blood pressure. It may even act to lower blood homocysteine levels. Include garlic in your meals regularly; it is best eaten raw, as cooking destroys some of the active components in it. Onion, leeks and spring onion all have similar properties to garlic, they are just not as strong. Ref.115.

Ginger has been used in India, Asia and Arabic countries as a medicine since ancient times. Modern research has shown that it helps to protect us against heart disease in a number of ways. Ginger helps to reduce inflammation in the body; you may be aware of its positive effects on arthritis and menstrual pain; these conditions are both stimulated by inflammation. By reducing inflammation, ginger is also able to inhibit the process of atherosclerosis in our arteries. Ginger is able to lower blood cholesterol and triglyceride levels, and because it is an antioxidant, it has the ability to prevent the oxidation of LDL "bad" cholesterol. Ref.116

Turmeric is becoming known as a wonder spice with the ability to prevent many diseases. It is a close relative of ginger, has an intensely yellow color and is the main ingredient in curry powder. The main benefits of turmeric are its strong antioxidant and anti-inflammatory actions. It is able to lower cholesterol levels and prevent the oxidation of LDL "bad" cholesterol. Turmeric also inhibits the accumulation of platelets in artery walls that have been damaged. This is good because it inhibits the formation of blood clots that can block arteries and lead to heart attacks and strokes. Research has also shown turmeric to exhibit

anti cancer effects, and inhibit the development of dementia. You
can find powdered turmeric in the supermarket, which you can use in
cooking. The fresh rhizome is often available in Asian grocery stores.
Ref.117.

6. Keep your homocysteine low

Vitamins B6, B12 and B9 (also called folic acid) are important to keep
your blood homocysteine levels low. Elevated homocysteine levels are a
major risk factor for heart disease because homocysteine has an abrasive
effect on the inner lining of our arteries, initiating inflammation and
atherosclerosis. It also makes the formation of blood clots more likely.
Folic acid, vitamin B12 and B6 all work together to keep homocysteine
levels low by helping to convert homocysteine into the amino acid
methionine.

Good sources of folic acid include oranges, avocados, spinach,
asparagus and any green leafy vegetable. Vitamin B6 is found in high
concentrations in bananas, salmon, chicken, potatoes and hazelnuts.
Good sources of vitamin B12 are salmon, mussels, crab, beef, chicken
and eggs. Betaine is another nutrient found in eggs which is needed to
keep homocysteine low.

If you have diagnosed elevated homocysteine levels in your blood, then
as well as eating these foods and drinking raw vegetable juices, you
will need to take a supplement of these vitamins. SAMe Boost capsules
contain vitamin B6, B12 and folic acid, plus other nutrients that help to
keep you homocysteine low.

Researchers at the Oregon Health and Science University in the US claim
that diets low in foods containing folate and carotenoids may be a "major
contributing factor" to the high rate of heart disease in men and women in
Central and Eastern Europe, compared with Western Europe, the US and
Asian countries. The researchers found substantially higher death rates

from cardiac disease among men and women, especially men between the ages of 30 and 50 years in Estonia, Hungary, Russia and Lithuania, which correlated with low intakes of folate and carotenoids in their diet. Ref.118 Carotenoids include beta carotene, lycopene, lutein and related compounds found mainly in brightly colored vegetables.

7. Improve your liver function

Approximately 80 percent of the cholesterol in your body was made in your liver, so it makes sense to take good care of it. If your liver is healthy, you should have a healthy cholesterol level. The amount of cholesterol we consume in our diet has very little effect on our blood cholesterol. The liver primarily converts excess calories from carbohydrates and sugar into cholesterol and triglycerides. Therefore, an excess of sugar and carbohydrate in the diet is one of the most common reasons why people develop a fatty liver. Trans fats are also responsible for the development of fatty liver disease; these are unnatural, twisted fats that our liver doesn't know what to do with. They can end up clogging your liver with unhealthy fat.

In modern times fatty liver disease has become extremely common, with approximately 20 percent of the population affected. You can find out if you have a fatty liver through the use of a liver ultrasound, a blood test called a liver function test, and just by observing if you carry excess weight on your abdominal area, especially the upper abdomen. If you need more specific information about fatty liver disease and how to reverse it, please see the book *"The Liver Cleansing Diet"*.

The liver is the cleanser and filter of the bloodstream; if you were to look at it under a microscope it really is built like a sieve. Your liver is responsible for keeping your bloodstream as clean as possible. Every chemical and toxin you are exposed to ultimately ends up in your liver. Whether it was something you inhaled, rubbed on to your skin, ate, or toxins that were generated in your own body; each of these are taken to your liver for detoxification. The liver attempts to change these toxins into a water-soluble form so that they can be excreted in watery fluids like the bile, urine, perspiration, and through the breath.

If you have a fatty liver, you surely have an excess of toxins stored there. Most toxic substances in our body are fat soluble, and an excess of fatty tissue in the liver will mean an excess of toxins. Many people with fatty liver disease have raised liver enzymes, this means that there is excessive inflammation in their liver, and as a consequence liver cells are being damaged. These inflammatory chemicals and toxins will spill out into the bloodstream and place a great deal of stress on the immune system. Remember that it is the liver that produces C-reactive protein when there is an excess of inflammation in the body; C-reactive protein is one of the biggest risk factors for heart disease we know of.

As you can see, one of the best ways to stem inflammation in your body, and take a burden off your immune system is to have healthy liver function. Avoiding trans fats, reducing your intake of sugar and carbohydrate, eating raw foods and consuming raw vegetable juices are all great ways to take care of your liver. Another great way to improve your liver health relatively quickly is to take a good liver tonic. A good liver tonic will increase the manufacture and flow of bile through your liver, thus taking toxins away with it, and increase the flow of bile out of your gallbladder; ensuring it stays healthy too. Look for the following ingredients in a liver tonic to make sure you are getting the best formula:

• St Mary's Thistle (Milk Thistle)
Also known as Silybum marianum, this herb promotes the excretion of bile through the liver, thus has a cleansing effect. It is very high in antioxidants; therefore it reduces the oxidation of cholesterol and prevents free radical damage in the body. Milk thistle also has the ability to repair and regenerate damaged liver cells.

• Dandelion Root (Taraxacum officinale)
This herb also promotes the flow of bile, therefore has a cleansing effect on a congested liver and gallbladder. Bile is one of the main ways we excrete cholesterol from our body, so if you can increase its flow, you will

be excreting more cholesterol. Dandelion root also has a mild laxative action, further helping cholesterol to be excreted.

• Globe artichoke (Cynara scolymus)
Globe artichoke stimulates the flow of bile; however it also has other direct cholesterol lowering actions. Clinical trials have shown it has the ability to reduce total and LDL "bad" cholesterol. Ref.119 Globe artichoke contains luteolin; a type of flavonoid which is a strong antioxidant. Luteolin has the ability to prevent the oxidation of LDL cholesterol, thus preventing it from doing harm to our arteries. Ref.120

• Taurine
This is a type of protein called an amino acid needed for various functions in the body. Taurine is involved in bile formation, detoxification of toxins called xenobiotics by the liver, stabilizing cell membranes and nerve cells. By helping to form bile, taurine assists with the removal of cholesterol from the body. Taurine also helps our arteries to be healthy, and can actually reverse some of the damage that smoking causes to them. According to Dr David J. Bouchier-Hayes, professor of surgery at the Royal College of Surgeons in Ireland, Beaumont Hospital, Dublin; "When blood vessels are exposed to cigarette smoke it causes the vessels to behave like a rigid pipe rather than a flexible tube, thus the vessels can't dilate in response to increased blood flow". This is referred to as endothelial dysfunction; it is one of the earliest signs of atherosclerosis. A study published in the journal *Circulation* showed that when smokers were given a taurine supplement, their blood vessels appeared to behave the same as non-smokers; taurine reversed the damage that smoking did to the arteries of the participants. Ref.121

The liver tonic Livatone contains the above four ingredients. Livatone Plus contains a high dose of Milk Thistle, plus vitamins and minerals.

If you wish to discuss liver tonics with a health consultant, please phone our Health Advisory Service on 623 334 3232.

8. Strengthen Your Immune System

Allergies, autoimmune diseases and infections all create a lot of inflammation in your body. People with autoimmune diseases such as systemic lupus erythematosus and rheumatoid arthritis are much more likely to have a heart attack than the general population. You are also more likely to have a heart attack during or soon after having an infection, such as the flu or pneumonia. Sometimes people with chronic, hidden infections such as gum disease, Helicobacter pylori or infection with cytomegalovirus are more prone to heart disease.

If you have a hyperstimulated, overworked immune system, it is likely that you have elevated levels of C-reactive protein. Immune cells also release a host of inflammation-promoting chemicals called inflammatory cytokines. Some of these include interferon, interlukin-6 and interleukin-10. As well as causing tissue damage, and the symptoms specific to various immune disorders, these chemicals all promote irritation and damage to your endothelium, or inner lining of your arteries.

What you can do to improve the function of your immune system

• Avoid eating foods you are allergic or intolerant to:
If you are continually exposed to something you are allergic or intolerant to, it acts like a poison in your body. Your immune system is continually fighting to counteract the effects of this food, and in the process produces a lot of chemicals that have damaging effects in your body. The foods that most commonly produce allergies/intolerances are dairy products, wheat, gluten, eggs, corn, tomatoes, soy and oranges. Possible symptoms you may experience if you have a food allergy/intolerance include:

- Abdominal bloating
- Skin rashes
- Foggy brain and poor concentration
- Fluid retention
- Headaches

- Joint or muscle aches and pains
- Irritable bowel syndrome
- Mood changes, anxiety or depression

An elimination diet that is guided by a naturopath or nutritionist is recommended to pinpoint your allergies. Many people with these symptoms have leaky gut syndrome, and this must be treated. There is more information about leaky gut syndrome, as well as a non-allergenic eating plan in our book *"The Ultimate Detox"*.

• Eat raw foods to nourish your immune system:

It is very important to eat fresh raw foods every day. Raw foods contain enzymes and nutrients which cooking may destroy and they take very little effort to digest. It is important to eat at least one raw vegetable salad each day; try to vary the vegetables you use and have a variety of different colored vegetables, as they each have different healing properties. Raw fruit is an excellent snack. As well as getting vitamins, minerals and antioxidants from fruit and vegetables to keep free radicals under control and prevent the oxidation of cholesterol, you obtain a lot of fiber from these foods, helping to remove cholesterol via your bowels.

• Use substances with infection fighting properties:

It is very important to keep infections under control, as they can do a great deal of harm to your body if allowed to flourish. Following a healthy diet free of sugar is important, as sugar feeds bacteria, yeast, fungi and parasites in our body. If you have a sweet tooth a healthy alternative to sugar is stevia. This is available in tablet form. Stevia can be added to tea and coffee, as well as used in cooking.

Vegetables in the cruciferous family (cabbage, broccoli, cauliflower, Brussels sprouts) all have infection fighting properties because they contain organic sulfur compounds. If you don't eat enough of these vegetables, you can obtain similar benefits by taking the supplement MSM. For more information about MSM please call our Health Advisory line on 623 334 3232. Garlic, onion, leeks, chives and spring onions are

all strong natural antibiotics. They are most potent when eaten raw.
Olive leaf extract contains the active ingredient oleuropein, which studies
have shown possesses antibacterial, antiviral and antifungal properties.
Olive leaf works well for a variety of infections, such as colds and flu,
respiratory infections, digestive and urinary infections. It is available in
capsule form.

• Do a bowel and liver detox:

Sometimes the greatest amount of toxins in your body are generated in
your digestive tract. Toxins created in your own body are referred to
as endotoxins. Bad habits such as eating when stressed or rushed, not
chewing properly and eating processed junk food can all create a toxic
state inside your gut. If you are prone to constipation the situation will
be even worse because toxins you are supposed to excrete will be re-
absorbed back into your bloodstream.

All the blood from your digestive tract travels to your liver via the hepatic
portal vein. If your intestines are toxic, then your liver will be before too
long. This scenario will place a great stress on the detoxification ability
of your liver, and will result in toxins spilling into your bloodstream.
Your immune system will be overworked, placing you at greater risk of
developing infections and allergies. Many of these toxic compounds
act as free radicals in the body and have direct inflammation inducing
actions. One of Dr Cabot's trained health consultants can guide you
through a thorough detox. Please call 623 334 32 32 to speak to our
friendly team. The book *"The Ultimate Detox"* contains a two week
deep cleansing eating plan. Intestinal Parasite Cleanse capsules contain
wormwood, black walnut, cloves and other herbs with anti-parasitic
properties in the digestive tract.

• Take vitamins and minerals to strengthen your immune system:

Our immune system needs plenty of vitamins and minerals to stay strong,
and with modern day diets and farming techniques, it is very easy to be
deficient in these. Selenium is a mineral that can be deficient in soil. It

is a powerful antioxidant, and has strong anti inflammatory and antiviral properties. Selenium is excellent for people who get repeated infections; have a long standing infection they can't get rid of; suffer with allergies, or an autoimmune disease. If your body is deficient in selenium, viruses entering it are more likely to mutate into a more harmful form. It is best to take selenium in its organic form called selenomethionine. An ideal dose would be 100-200mcg per day. Selenium works best when it is combined with vitamin E, zinc and vitamin C. You can find selenium in tablet form or as a designer energy powder.

As well as helping to fight infections, vitamin C and bioflavonoids have an anti allergic effect in our body; they reduce the amount of histamine released from white blood cells. If you suffer with allergies such as hayfever, sinusitis or eczema, it is strongly recommended that you take a good vitamin C supplement.

9. Manage Your Stress

We all know that stress is bad for our health. You can have a perfect diet and exercise regularly, yet if stress is a big part of your life you are still likely to get sick. The stress hormones adrenalin and cortisol promote inflammation in our bodies, cause us to gain weight, make us more likely to develop Syndrome X and suppress our immune system. Ongoing stress usually leads to depression, and depressed people are more likely to suffer with heart disease. These are mostly consequences of long term stress; acute stress reactions can be even more damaging.

Not all heart attacks occur as a result of fatty plaques deposited in the artery walls; it is possible to have a heart attack even if you have healthy arteries. Sometimes there is a spasm of the coronary arteries which reduces or stops blood flow through these arteries that lead to the heart. Spasm of the coronary arteries can lead to chest pain, and it may even cause a fatal heart attack.

Can you die of a broken heart?

It seems like mom was wrong, and you can in fact die of a broken heart. Extreme sadness, sudden fright and other intense negative emotions can result in symptoms of a heart attack, and in susceptible people will actually cause a heart attack. A study published in the *New England Journal of Medicine* examined 19 patients who had very recently had a traumatic experience; these patients had been admitted to hospital with heart attack like symptoms. These patients were found to have more than seven times the normal levels of the stress hormones adrenalin and dopamine in their bloodstream. These hormones regulate heart rate and blood pressure. Ref.122 Mental stress can impair the normal rhythm of the heart and cause impaired blood flow to the heart muscle.

Several studies have shown that workplace stress and pressure place people at greater risk of having a heart attack. This is especially so if the person does not feel they have any control over their circumstances at work. Heart attacks are said to be more common on Monday mornings!

Too little sleep is very bad for your heart also, as not getting enough sleep is a stress on your body. Researchers at Brigham and Women's Hospital in Boston, USA found that women who reported sleeping five hours or less per night were 45 percent more likely to have heart problems than women who sleep eight hours per night. Ref.123

Think happy thoughts

Just as negative emotions impair heart function, pleasant, relaxing emotions have a positive effect on the heart. It is very important to take time out of your day, even if it is only ten minutes to do something that makes you happy. Our lives can be busy and stressful, leaving no time for fun and relaxation. Many studies have shown meditation, yoga and breathing exercises to have very positive effects on overall health. By slowing down your breathing you can lower your blood pressure.

Laughter and love can help to keep our heart strong and healthy. Dr Michael Miller, of the University of Maryland School of Medicine in Baltimore, USA showed two movies to 20 healthy volunteers; one stressful and one humorous. He specifically looked at the endothelium, or inner lining of the arteries of the volunteers. Dr Miller found that blood flow decreased 35 percent during the stressful movie, and increased 22 percent during laughter. He concluded that "Laughter might be almost as helpful as exercise" to our heart, and recommended 15 minutes of laughter each day. Ref.124

Several studies have shown that feeling love helps people to live longer, healthier lives. A 2002 Australian National Heart Foundation study showed that social isolation and lack of group support are as important as high cholesterol, high blood pressure and smoking in people with heart disease. A study of 1000 Israeli men with heart disease found that men who felt loved by their wives were 50 percent less likely to experience angina and heart attacks than those with problematic relationships. According to Professor Marc Cohen, who spoke at the International Conference on Health, Ageing and Longevity in Brisbane, Australia in 2005, it is not just romantic love that helps to keep us healthy. It can be love for anyone or anything that makes you feel as though time has stopped. Even hobbies that we love, and become totally immersed in are beneficial. Ref.125

Magnesium is a mineral with many benefits to the cardiovascular system. It is very important for helping to maintain a normal heart rhythm and normal blood pressure. Magnesium has a relaxing effect on the muscles and nerves of the body thus can relax the coronary arteries and reduce the chance of spasms. Magnesium is excellent for highly stressed people, as it helps the body to cope with stress, and helps you to feel calmer. If there is a lot of stress in your life that is unavoidable, you need to take supplemental magnesium. When we are stressed, our body uses up greater amounts of magnesium, so we can easily become deficient in this mineral. A high dietary intake of fat and calcium make you more likely to become magnesium deficient. Interestingly, magnesium deficiency increases the release of the stress hormones adrenaline and noradrenaline, making you feel even more wound up. A lack of magnesium makes you more susceptible to high blood pressure and irregular heart rhythms called arrhythmias. Ref. 126 Those who are magnesium deficient are at increased risk of sudden cardiac death, coronary artery spasm and arrhythmia.

Constructive ways to beat stress

There is no way to eliminate stress from our lives entirely, and small amounts are actually good for providing motivation and stimulating creativity. To make sure stress doesn't take control of your life and health, try to follow these tips:

- Make the time to do simple things you enjoy. This could be listening to your favorite music, reading a good book, phoning a friend or meeting them for lunch.

- Spend time with people who make you laugh, and watch comedies.

- Make sure you get enough sleep. If you are chronically tired, every difficulty will be harder to cope with.

- Exercise. It is impossible to be thinking about your problems if you are flat out exercising.

- If something is bothering you, talk about it to a friend or family member you trust.

- Take a holiday each year. You don't have to go far; just a change in scenery and routine can do wonders for restoring motivation.

- Find something in life you are passionate about and be involved in it regularly. Life has so many things to offer, there is never a reason to feel bored.

- Remember to be grateful for all the wonderful people and things in your life.

- Having a regular massage is a great way to release tension from your body.

- Learn meditation, yoga or tai chi. Stress management techniques like this can reduce your risk of heart disease by 50 percent. Ref.127

- Breath slowly and deeply. Often when we are stressed we take shallow breaths or hold our breath for short periods of time.

10. Exercise Is Vital

We all know that exercise is good for us, but you may not know just how much it can save your life. If someone could bottle the positive effects exercise has on our bodies and sell it as a drug, they would make a fortune because we'd all be taking it! Interestingly enough there was a weight loss supplement on the American market called "Exercise in a Bottle"; the US Federal Trade Commission has permanently banned the manufacturer of this supplement from marketing products for weight loss because of false and unsubstantiated claims made about this supplement. There's nothing like the real thing!

Exercise has the following benefits for your heart:

- It makes your heart muscle stronger, so that it can pump more blood with less effort.

- It helps you maintain a healthy weight by speeding up your metabolism and increasing your muscle mass.

- Reduces your chance of having high blood pressure.

- Strengthens your immune system and improves your ability to fight off infections.

- Exercise reduces LDL "bad" cholesterol and triglycerides, and is one of the few ways you can increase your HDL "good" cholesterol.

- It improves glucose tolerance, thus reduces your chance of developing Syndrome X and diabetes.

- Exercise helps you cope with stress and reduces anxiety and depression. It reduces tension, anger and fatigue, and helps to lift your spirits. Ref.128

- Exercise improves your self esteem and makes you more motivated to eat well and look after yourself well.

- It causes your artery walls to release nitric oxide, which dilates your blood vessels, improving blood flow; reducing inflammation of the artery walls and reducing the tendency of blood clots to form in the arteries.

- Exercise makes you smarter! Yes it's true; studies have shown that exercise helps thinking and decision making abilities, and speeds up brain activity. Ref.129

- It helps you to live longer. Ref.130

Clearly exercise is one of the easiest, least expensive things you can do to reduce your risk of heart disease. An ideal amount of exercise would be 30 to 60 minutes most days of the week. If you can't fit it all in one go, you can split this into two or three sessions. For example, two fifteen minute walks would be just as good. If you don't have time for formal exercise, you can still stay active by gardening, doing vigorous housework, walking to the shops instead of driving, taking the stairs instead of the lift, going out dancing, or having energetic sex. Find some way to be more active; it will be well worth it.

If you have diagnosed heart disease it is vital that you check with your doctor before starting an exercise program.

Other factors that have been found to influence the development of heart disease.

Air pollution causes heart disease

The burning of fossil fuels is thought to increase your risk of heart disease. Tiny airborne particles that are released from power stations, motor vehicles, burning wood and steel and cement plants are light and can travel 2000 to 3000 kilometers in air currents. According to Markus Amann, from the International Institute for Applied Systems Analysis, these particles cause heart disease by inflaming the heart membranes. The United Nation's Economic Commission for Europe is planning to set up a team to investigate the problem. Ref.131

Lack of sunlight raises your cholesterol

When our skin is exposed to sunlight, the cholesterol in our skin is converted into hormone precursors, which are then converted into vitamin D and testosterone. The cholesterol in your bloodstream then moves into your skin to replace what was lost. Therefore, regularly getting small amounts of sunlight on your skin can help to keep your cholesterol down, your bones strong, and your libido healthy, through increased testosterone production. Ref.132 This may be one of the reasons why shift workers have twice the rate of heart disease of the general population. Ref.133

Too much iron can give you a heart attack

Iron is an essential mineral in our body that is mainly required for the transport of oxygen in the bloodstream. However, too much iron can do a lot of damage in your body. Iron has an oxidizing effect in our body, and if you have too much of it, it acts as a free radical. Iron can oxidize the cholesterol in your bloodstream, turning it into a much more harmful state.

Excess iron can also cause damage to the inner lining of your arteries (endothelium), making you more likely to develop atherosclerosis. It seems that too much iron interferes with the action of nitric oxide. This is a substance produced by our artery walls that dilates blood vessels, and has an anti inflammatory effect on the arteries. Ref.134 If you have some risk factors for heart disease, such as high cholesterol, a fatty liver or diabetes, it is very important for you to have a blood test for iron. Menstruation in women, and blood donations by men, are considered to offer protection against heart disease because of the loss of iron. One study published in the *British Medical Journal* found that male blood donors have an 86 percent lower chance of having a heart attack than non-donors. Ref.135

Sleep apnea

Severe sleep apnea is a bigger risk to your heart than smoking or high blood pressure. If left untreated, sleep apnea can make you five times more likely to have a heart attack. Sleep apnea is where the muscles of the back of the throat and tongue relax so much during sleep that they collapse and block the airways. When this happens a person stops breathing. After a few seconds to a minute, the brain detects that not enough oxygen is getting into the body. The brain then forces you awake so that you can take a breath. Typically this recurs several times each night. The common scenario is that a person will be snoring during their sleep, stop breathing momentarily, and then start choking or coughing. They fall back asleep straight away and start snoring again.

People who suffer with sleep apnea are usually very sleepy during the day and experience poor concentration and irritability. The most common causes of this condition are obesity, alcohol consumption in the evening and nasal congestion. Not everyone who snores has sleep apnea. This condition is diagnosed via an overnight sleep study, whereby you spend a night at a hospital and electrodes are taped to various parts of your body to monitor sleep quality and breathing.

Sleep apnea can often be totally cured with diet and lifestyle changes such as losing weight, reducing alcohol intake, especially in the evening, and treating excessive mucus congestion in the sinuses and respiratory tract. Sleeping on your side rather than back usually helps too. More severe cases require the use of a CPAP (nasal Continuous Positive Airway Pressure) machine. This is a nasal mask worn at night which pumps air into your upper airway to keep it open. This method is very effective but it can be difficult to get used to. Treatment with a CPCP machine removes the risk of heart disease incurred by sleep apnea.

Chapter Thirteen

THE HEART-SAVING DIET IN A NUTSHELL

• Don't eat too much carbohydrate.
Grains, sugar and starches promote high cholesterol, weight gain and make you more likely to develop diabetes. If you are at risk of heart disease you will need to avoid sugar and strictly limit your intake of bread, pasta, rice, breakfast cereals, potatoes, rice, bananas and all foods containing flour. The book *"Can't Lose Weight? Unlock The Secrets That Keep You Fat"* contains a delicious, easy to follow low carbohydrate eating plan.

• Avoid trans fatty acids.
These are labeled on foods as "hydrogenated vegetable oil", "partially hydrogenated vegetable oil" or "vegetable fat". These are man made,

chemically altered fats that are formed when a liquid vegetable oil is turned into a solid, such as in margarine. They are also present in many cooking oils that have been extracted using heat. Trans fats raise LDL "bad" cholesterol, lower HDL "good" cholesterol and promote inflammation in your body. They promote the development of insulin resistance (Syndrome X), and in this way make you fat. The best fats to eat are those labeled "cold pressed" or "extra virgin", as well as virgin coconut fat, butter and ghee. Saturated fats are not as bad for you as the media claim. Foods such as eggs, red meat and butter have been part of the human diet for many generations, at a time when heart disease was rare. Moderate amounts of saturated fat in the diet are not a problem in healthy individuals. There are many cases of vegans, who eat no animal products yet have high cholesterol.

• Don't smoke cigarettes.
Hundreds of toxic chemicals are present in cigarettes which inflame and damage the artery walls. This promotes high blood pressure and the development of fatty deposits on the artery walls. Cigarettes are a major source of free radicals, contributing to inflammation in the body. Nicotine stimulates the production of adrenaline, which increases your heart rate and blood pressure.

• Look after your liver.
The liver is the major site of cholesterol production, therefore if it is kept healthy; you should not have a cholesterol problem. Approximately 20 percent of Americans have a fatty liver, whereby fatty tissue replaces normal liver cells, severely compromising liver function. Unless you work on improving your liver function, you will not be able to achieve a healthy cholesterol level.

• Eat good fats.
Monounsaturated and polyunsaturated fats help to keep your cholesterol levels in check. Suitable foods to include in your diet are olive oil, avocados and raw nuts and seeds. Omega 3 fats are especially beneficial for the heart, and are found in fish, walnuts, ground flaxseeds and flaxseed oil. Ground flaxseeds should be kept in the freezer, and can be

found combined with ground almonds and sunflower seeds, as "LSA".

• Stress less.

Stress is a major contributor to the development of many diseases, but particularly heart disease. Having chronically elevated stress hormones running through your bloodstream promotes inflammation and weakens your immune system. It is important to make time to do things you enjoy, and surround yourself with a network of people you love.

• Exercise is a must.

It will help to keep your weight down, greatly reduce the risk of Syndrome X and diabetes and it is an excellent stress buster. Exercise helps to keep your LDL "bad" cholesterol and triglycerides down, and is one of the few ways to raise your levels of HDL "good" cholesterol.

• Get lots of antioxidants into your diet.

It is not cholesterol, but rather oxidized cholesterol that does the harm to your arteries. You need plenty of antioxidants to prevent the cholesterol in your body from oxidizing. You can do this by ensuring you get the recommended five servings of vegetables and two servings of fruit each day. Making your own raw vegetable juices regularly is a sure way of getting enough fruit and veggies. Antioxidants are also found in raw nuts and seeds, legumes, green tea, red wine and dark chocolate.

Chapter Fourteen

HEART HEALTHY RECIPES

The vegetable juices below work in different ways to help protect you against heart disease. Vegetable juices are a concentrated source of vitamins, minerals, enzymes and phyto chemicals, all helping to keep your cardiovascular system healthy. Juices are an easy and tasty way of upping your fruit and vegetable intake. Vegetable juices are powerful antioxidants, and in this way help to keep the inner lining of your blood vessels healthy, and prevent the oxidation of cholesterol in your body. Each juice below works on a different principle, all helping to lower your risk of heart disease. It is best to make each of these juices regularly, concentrating on your particular risk factors. It is recommended you consume these juices immediately after you make them. However, it is possible to squeeze a little lemon juice into the vegetable juice, to act as a preservative, and then keep it refrigerated for a maximum of one day.

CHOLESTEROL LOWERING AND ANTIOXIDANT JUICE

½ cup blueberries
½ cup black grapes
1 slice red onion
2 stalks celery
Dilute with ½ cup strong green tea

Elevated LDL cholesterol is a risk factor for heart disease. However, if your cholesterol becomes oxidized, due to a lack of antioxidants in your diet, or the consumption of fried, processed foods, it becomes especially harmful.
Blueberries contain the natural compound pterostilbene, which acts to lower LDL cholesterol. Grapes contain the antioxidant resveratrol, which helps to prevent the oxidation of cholesterol, and keeps the arteries healthy. Onions contain the powerful antioxidant quercetin. Celery acts as a natural diuretic, helping to keep blood pressure normal. Green tea contains powerful antioxidants that prevent the oxidation of cholesterol, reduce inflammation in the arteries, and green tea has a direct cholesterol lowering effect.

INFLAMMATION FIGHTER

5cm slice pineapple
1cm fresh ginger root
1 grapefruit – including the pith
1 carrot
2 stalks celery

People with too much inflammation in their bodies often have elevated blood levels of C-reactive protein. This is a major risk factor for heart disease. Excess inflammation causes damage to the inner lining of the arteries.

Pineapple is a strong natural anti-inflammatory. Ginger reduces inflammation in the body, improves circulation and helps to prevent the oxidation of LDL "bad" cholesterol. Grapefruit contains organic salicylic acid which is a natural anti-inflammatory. Carrot and celery both contain phthalides, which inhibit inflammation.

INFECTION FIGHTER

1 clove garlic
1 slice red onion
2 red radishes
¼ pineapple
1 ripe tomato
½ lemon

Hidden chronic infections are strongly linked to an increased risk of heart disease.

Garlic and onion are powerful natural antibiotics. Radishes are cleansing, helping to clear the bloodstream of toxins. Pineapple has strong mucus fighting properties, helping to clear respiratory infections in particular. Tomatoes contain natural antiseptic properties. Lemon helps to break up mucus and is a natural antiseptic.

LIVER TONIC JUICE

1 handful chicory - use kale if you cannot find chicory
1 handful collard
1 carrot
2 stalks celery
½ beetroot
½ broccoli floweret

Approximately 80 percent of the cholesterol in your body is manufactured in your liver. It is essential to have a healthy liver if you want to reduce your risk of heart disease. Typically people with a fatty liver have elevated levels of LDL "bad" cholesterol and triglycerides.

Chicory and collard are bitter vegetables that stimulate the flow of bile, therefore have a flushing effect on the liver and gallbladder. Carrot and celery are high in minerals and have a gentle cleansing effect on the liver. Beetroot is a strong liver detoxifier. Broccoli is high in organic sulfur compounds, needed for the enzymes involved in liver detoxification.

HEALTHY BOWEL JUICE

2 handfuls of chicory or collard
1 green apple, including the skin
1 pear, including the skin
1 orange – pith included
2 radishes

The major route of excretion of cholesterol from the body is via the bowels. A high intake of fiber binds to cholesterol in the intestines and carries it out of the body.

Chicory and collard are bitter vegetables that stimulate bile flow; bile is the body's natural laxative. Apples and oranges are high in pectin, which is a soluble fiber; pears are one of the highest fiber fruits. Radishes stimulate the liver and gallbladder, helping to keep the bowels regular.

HOMOCYSTEINE LOWERING JUICE

5 asparagus spears

1 bunch English spinach
1 orange – pith included
1 carrot

Homocysteine is a type of protein that if elevated in the bloodstream is a major risk factor for heart disease. Ensuring you have an adequate intake of folic acid, vitamin B6 and vitamin B12 is one of the best ways to keep your homocysteine levels low.

Asparagus, spinach and oranges are the richest sources of folic acid. Carrot contains some B vitamins, and helps to keep the mucous membranes of the digestive tract healthy. Vitamins B6 and B12 are found in greatest amounts in animal foods such as chicken, seafood, beef and eggs.

BLOOD SUGAR BALANCING JUICE

½ cup chopped fennel
½ cup green beans
½ broccoli floweret

Poor glucose tolerance, insulin resistance and Syndrome X are all terms used to describe poor blood sugar control and inefficient action of the hormone insulin. This scenario places people at increased risk of diabetes, obesity, and high cholesterol levels.
Fennel, green beans and broccoli all act to assist the action of insulin, and keep blood sugar levels stable.

HEART SAVING SOUP

Ingredients
2 cups red kidney beans
3 cups water

3 tablespoons red wine (optional)
2 onions, chopped
3 cloves garlic, crushed (optional)
1 Tbsp olive oil
3 carrots, chopped
2 stalks celery, chopped
1 red capsicum, chopped
1 bunch asparagus, chopped
2 bay leaves
15oz tomato paste
½ tsp cumin
1 tsp turmeric
½ tsp black pepper
½ tsp dried oregano
1 tsp sea salt
2 Tbsp fresh parsley, chopped
2 Tbsp red lentils

Method
Place the beans in a large saucepan, cover with water and leave to soak overnight. Discard the soaking water, rinse the beans and place them in a large soup pot. Place the 8 cups of water in the pot, bring the beans to the boil, put the lid on and reduce the heat to simmer.
In a large saucepan sauté the onion and garlic in the olive oil for 3 minutes. Add the carrots, celery, capsicum and asparagus. Sauté until the mixture has cooked slightly; approximately 8 minutes. Add the vegetable mixture to the beans, then add all remaining ingredients except the fresh parsley. Simmer on a low heat until the beans are soft. Stir in the fresh parsley; cook a further 2 minutes, and then serve with a salad.

Benefits of the Heart Saving Soup

Vegetables are high in antioxidants, which reduce inflammation and prevent the oxidation of cholesterol.

All legumes, including navy beans and red lentils are an excellent source of fiber, and in particular soluble fiber. This binds with cholesterol in the intestines and carries it out of the body in bowel movements.

Red wine contains the powerful antioxidant resveratrol. Regular red wine consumption may significantly reduce your risk of heart disease.

Extra virgin olive oil is the preferred choice for cooking, as it can tolerate high temperatures without becoming damaged. Olive oil is high in monounsaturated fat and helps to keep LDL "bad" cholesterol down, while increasing HDL "good" cholesterol.

Garlic and onion contain powerful infection fighting properties, helping to keep the immune system strong.

Tomato paste is a concentrated source of the antioxidant lycopene. Fat, such as olive oil increases the absorption of lycopene from tomatoes.

Spices such as cumin, turmeric and oregano are high in antioxidants that help to prevent the oxidation of cholesterol.

Essential Shopping List to Protect Your Heart

These are the foods you must have in your pantry and fridge to protect yourself against heart disease.

Raw nuts. All nuts must be unsalted and not roasted. Suitable varieties include almonds, Brazil nuts, pine nuts, walnuts, pecans, macadamia nuts, pistachios, hazelnuts and cashews. Walnuts and almonds are especially beneficial. Nuts are an excellent source of fiber and beneficial fats. They have a low GI, therefore are excellent for helping to prevent diabetes. Nuts make an ideal snack, or they can be added to salads. A handful a day is the recommended quantity.

Raw seeds. All seeds must be unsalted and not roasted. Suitable varieties include sunflower seeds, pepitas (pumpkin seeds), sesame seeds and linseeds. These may be added to salads or used as a snack. Linseeds need to be ground in a coffee grinder or food processor. They can be added to cereal, smoothies, yogurt, or sprinkled over fruit.

Fats and oils. Olive oil may be used as a dressing over salad or vegetables, either on its own, or combined with vinegar, lemon or lime juice. Olive oil may be used for cooking.
Flaxseed oil should never be heated; it can only be used cold as a salad dressing, or added to smoothies.
Virgin, unrefined coconut fat has many health benefits, and it is highly stable, thus may be used for cooking. Suitable brands include Nutiva, Tropical Traditions and Garden of Life.
Small amounts of butter and ghee may be used; preferably they would be organic.

Fish. This is best included in your diet four times a week. Fresh or canned fish may be used; suitable varieties include sardines, salmon, mackerel, tuna, herring and trout. Fresh prawns, crab and other shellfish may also be consumed.

Eggs. You may eat eggs every day if you like. Free range, organic or omega 3 eggs are preferable. The best cooking methods are boiling and poaching.

Chicken. Free range or organic chicken is best. Chicken is an excellent source of protein for those trying to lose weight and reduce their carbohydrate intake.

Red meat. Lean beef, veal, lamb, pork and game meat can be eaten a few times a week. Preferably this would be organic and pasture fed, not grain fed. Pasture fed meat is higher in omega 3 fats. Preferable cooking methods are boiling, roasting or stir frying.

Fruit and vegetables. All fruit and vegetables should be as fresh as possible. Try to buy produce that is in season and has been grown locally. Aim to have at least five vegetables and two pieces of fruit each day. Bananas and potatoes should be limited if you are overweight and limiting your carbohydrate intake.

Legumes. Suitable varieties include chick peas, kidney beans, black beans, pinto beans, navy beans, Lima beans, black eyed peas, lentils and others. These can be bought dried; this requires soaking and boiling, or tinned and ready to use. Legumes are an excellent source of fiber, which helps to carry cholesterol out of the body in bowel movements. Aim to consume ½ cup three times a week. They can be added to salads, stews, soups and casseroles.

Spreads and dips. The following are all suitable to use as alternatives to margarine or butter: avocado, hummus, baba ganoush, tahini, nut butter/spread (eg. peanut, almond, cashew, hazelnut or macadamia paste), tomato paste.

Red wine. One glass daily with a meal for women and two glasses for men is an ideal quantity. It is best to have at least three alcohol free days per week.

Dark chocolate. A maximum of 100 grams per day is recommended. Look for chocolate that contains between 70 and 85 percent cocoa solids.

Green tea. Ideally you would drink three cups a day. If you do not like the taste of green tea, purchase a variety that has been flavored with other herbs such as mint or lemon. Oolong tea is also highly beneficial.

Garlic and onion. These are best eaten raw, as cooking can damage some of the infection fighting properties they contain.

Spices. Ginger, turmeric, fenugreek, rosemary, cumin and others. Most spices have natural antibiotic actions and they are high in antioxidants, helping to reduce inflammation in your body. Many of them are helpful for stabilizing blood sugar levels, thus are good for people with Syndrome X and diabetes. Using spices in your cooking reduces the need for salt. Small amounts of sea salt can be used, unless you have high blood pressure and are sensitive to salt.

Grains. These are all fairly high in carbohydrate and should be limited. Oats and barley are high in soluble fiber and have cholesterol lowering properties. Rolled oats are best used to make porridge; barley can be added to soups, and some bread contains added barley. Bread should be limited, and only that with a low GI or made of stone ground flour should be used.

Stevia. This can be obtained in tablet form. Stevia is an ideal natural, non-calorie sweetener to use in place of sugar in tea, coffee and cooking.

Glossary

Angina pectoris: Pain that is experienced in the chest, but may radiate to the arms or jaw as a result of inadequate blood supply to the heart. Pain is often brought on by exertion.

Arrhythmia: An abnormal heart rhythm. The heart may beat too fast (tachycardia) or too slow (bradycardia), or be irregular. This can sometimes lead to a heart attack.

Atherosclerosis: Is also called arteriosclerosis, and refers to a hardening of the arteries. Cholesterol containing plaque forms in the artery walls, causing a narrowing and loss of elasticity in the arteries.

Cardiovascular disease: Disease that affects the heart and blood vessels, usually as a result of atherosclerosis. It usually refers to heart attack, stroke and congestive heart failure.

Cerebrovascular disease: Disease of the blood vessels that supply the brain. It usually refers to Transient Ischemic Attack (TIA) and stroke.

Congestive heart failure: A disease of the heart where it has weakened and lost the ability to pump blood around the body. Symptoms include fluid retention, weakness, shortness of breath and inability to exercise.

Coronary heart disease: Heart disease that results from blockage of the coronary arteries, which lead to the heart because of atherosclerosis. The blockage may eventually lead to a heart attack.

Creatine kinase (CK): This is an enzyme found mainly in the heart, brain and skeletal muscles. If a blood test shows this enzyme to be elevated, it usually means the cells where it is found have been injured or damaged. CK can be raised following a heart attack or the breakdown of skeletal muscle cells, which is a possible side effect of statin drugs (rhabdomyolysis).

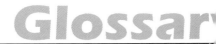

Cytokine: A messenger chemical made by one cell that affects the behavior of other cells.

Embolus: A blood clot that travels through the bloodstream and eventually lodges in a small blood vessel, blocking circulation.

Endothelium: A layer of cells that forms the inner lining of arteries and other cavities of the body. Healthy endothelial cells in our arteries promote dilation and inhibit platelets from clumping together.

Fatty acid: The building blocks of fats and oils. Three fatty acids joined together with glycerol form a triglyceride.

Foam cell: Fat filled macrophages that are found in fatty plaques on artery walls. To a lesser extent fat filled smooth muscle cells in fatty plaques are also called foam cells.

Free radical: An atom or group of atoms that have at least one unpaired electron. This makes it unstable and highly reactive. Free radicals can cause damage to DNA, cell membranes, fats and other substances in the body.

Homocysteine: A sulfur containing amino acid. It is an intermediate product in the metabolism of the amino acid methionine. Elevated blood levels of homocysteine are a major risk factor for heart disease.

Impaired glucose tolerance: A metabolic state whereby blood sugar levels are higher than normal, but not high enough to be considered diabetes. It usually means a blood sugar level between 110mg/dL and 124mg/dL.

Insulin resistance: Impaired response to the hormone insulin. There is a loss of sensitivity to insulin, which results in increased blood levels of this hormone. Insulin resistance is also referred to as Syndrome X and metabolic syndrome.

Ischemia: A low oxygen state, usually because of a lack of blood to a tissue or organ.

Lipids: Types of fats, for example cholesterol, triglycerides, phospholipids.

Lipoproteins: Particles that are a combination of fat and protein. They are used to transport fat and cholesterol around the bloodstream. HDL and LDL are examples of lipoproteins.

Leukocyte: A general term for a white blood cell.

Lymphocyte: A white blood cell. There are two types: T cells (responsible for cell-mediated immunity) and B cells (responsible for producing antibodies).

Macrophage: A type of white blood cell that engulfs foreign substances such as bacteria, tumor cells and other debris.

Methyl group: This is a molecule of one carbon atom with 3 hydrogen atoms attached to it. It is often represented as –CH3. Vitamin B6 and folic acid donate methyl groups to homocysteine, in order to convert it back into methionine.

Monocyte: A type of white blood cell that circulates in the blood. When it enters tissues it changes into a macrophage.

Myocardial infarction: This is commonly referred to as a heart attack.

Myopathy: Any disease involving the muscles.

Phospholipids: A type of fat where two fatty acids and phosphoric acid are attacked to a glycerol molecule. Phospholipids form cell membranes.

Serum: The liquid part of blood, or that part without the blood cells.

Stroke: Also called a cerebrovascular accident (CVA) and involves the

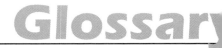

sudden death of some brain cells due to a lack of oxygen. A stroke can be ischemic, where blood flow is impaired because of a clot, or hemorrhagic, where a blood vessel in the brain ruptures.

Thrombus: A blood clot that forms inside a blood vessel or in a cavity of the heart.

Trans fatty acid: A fat produced by the partial hydrogenation of vegetable oil, present in hardened vegetable fat such as some margarines, cookies and many fried foods. Rather than the natural cis structure, the fatty acid chain possesses a trans structure.

Transient ischemic attack (TIA): Sometimes referred to as a mini stroke, this is a temporary disturbance of blood supply to a part of the brain. There is a sudden and brief disruption to brain function.

Triglycerides: Three fatty acids attached to a glycerol molecule. These are the major type of fat in our diet, and are also produced by our body. Most body fat is triglycerides.

References

1. American Heart Association.
2. Alpert PT. New and emerging theories of cardiovascular disease: infection and elevated iron. Biol Res Nurs. 2004 Jul;6(1):3-10.
3. vitamincfoundation.org
4. Drug Makers Race to Cash in on Fight against Fat NY Times April 3, 2005.
5. American Heart Association.
6. (Almost) Everything You Need To Know About Statin Drugs. Center For Medical Consumers.
7. American Journal of Clinical Nutrition. 1967 20:462-475
8. The Lancet. 14 November 1987
9. Fat Substitute Is Pushed Out Of the Kitchen. New York Times, Feb 13, 2005
10. Booyens J, Louwrens CC, Katzeff IE. The role of unnatural dietary trans and cis unsaturated fatty acids in the epidemiology of coronary artery disease. Med Hypotheses 1988; 25:175-182.
11. Mensink RPM, Katan MB. Effect of dietary trans fatty acids on high density and low-density lipoprotein cholesterol levels in healthy subjects. N Engl J Med 1990; 323:439-45.
12. Harvard School of Public Health.
13. Hu FB, Stampfer MJ, Manson JE, et al. Dietary fat intake and the risk of coronary heart disease in women. N Engl J Med 1997; 337:1491 1499
14. Fat Substitute Is Pushed Out of the Kitchen. New York Times, Feb 13, 2005
15. Carr MC et al. Abdominal Obesity and Dyslipidemia in the Metabolic Syndrome: Importance of Type 2 Diabetes and Familial Hyperlipidemia in Coronary Artery Disease Risk. Journal of Clinical Endocrinology and Metabolism 2004, 89(6)
16. Friedlander Y. Familial clustering of coronary heart disease: a review of its significance and role as a risk factor for the disease. In: Goldbourt U, de Faire U, Berg K editors. Genetic factors in coronary heart disease. Hingham Mass: Kluwer Academic Publishers. 1994:37 53

17. Breslow JL. Genetics of lipoprotein abnormalities associated with coronary artery disease susceptibility. Annu Rev Genet. 2000;34:233 254.

18. Hueston, William J., Pearson, William S., Subclinical Hypothyroidism and the Risk of Hypercholesterolemia. Annuals of Family Medicine 2:351-355 (2004)

19. Feld S, Dickey RA. An Association Between Varying Degrees of Hypothyroidism and Hypercholesterolemia in Women: The Thyroid Cholesterol Connection. Prev Cardiol. 2001 Autumn;4(4):179-182

20. Platzer C, et al. Catecholamines trigger IL-10 release in acute systemic stress reaction by direct stimulation of its promoter/enhancer activity in monocytic cells. J Neuroimmunol. 2000 Jun 1;105(1):31-8.

21. Liao J, et al. Role of epinephrine in TNF and IL-6 production from isolated perfused rat liver. Am J Physiol. 1995 Apr;268(4 Pt 2):R896 901

22. Ekelund L G et al. Physical fitness as a predictor of cardiovascular mortality in asymptomatic North American men. The Lipid Research Clinics mortality follow-up study. The New England Journal of Medicine 1988;319:1379-84

23. Craig WE, Palomaki GE, Haddow JE. Cigarette smoking and serum lipid and lipoprotein concentrations: an analysis of published data. British Medical Journal 1989;298:784-788.

24. Australian Heart Foundation

25. Australian Heart Foundation

26. Heart Research Foundation of Sacramento.

27. Beatrice A. Golomb, MD PhD on Statin Drugs, March 7, 2002

28. Gaist D. et al. Neurology 2002 May 14;58(9):1321-2.

29. JAMA 1996 Jan 3;275(1):55-60

30. Sacks, et. al. N Eng J Med 1996;385:1001-1009

31. American Heart Association.

32. Muldoon MF et. al. Am J Med 2000 May;108(7):538-46

33. Wagstaff LR, Mitton MW, McLendon Arvik B, Doraiswamy PM. Statin-Associated Memory Loss: Analysis of 60 Case Reports and Review of the Literature. Pharmacotherapy 2003;23(7):871-880

34. Tan ZS, et al. Plasma total cholesterol level as a risk factor for Alzheimer's disease: the Framingham study. Arch Intern Med

2003;163:1053-1057

35. Kash Rizvi, John P Hampson, John N Harvey. Do lipid lowering drugs cause erectile dysfunction? A systematic review. Family Practice Vol. 19, No. 1, 95-98

36. Azzarito C, Boiardi L, Vergoni W, Zini M, Portioli I. Testicular function in hypercholesterolemic male patients during prolonged simvastatin treatment. Horm Metab Res 1996;28:193-8

37. Smals AG, Weusten JJ, Benraad TJ, Kloppenborg PW. The HMG CoA reductase-inhibitor simvastatin suppresses human testicular testosterone synthesis in vitro by a selective inhibitory effect on 17 ketosteroid-oxidoreductase enzyme activity. J Steroid Biochem Mol Biol 1991;38:465-8

38. Kash Rizvi, John P Hampson, John N Harvey. Do lipid lowering drugs cause erectile dysfunction? A systematic review. Family Practice Vol. 19, No. 1, 95-98

39. Cholesterol lowering drugs linked to cataracts. Kirksville College of Osteopathic Medicine

40. Letter to the FDA shows that Crestor has higher rates of rhabdomyolysis compared to other statins. March 10, 2005. www.citizen.org

41. La Rosa, John C. et al, Intensive Lipid Lowering With Atorvastatin in Patients with Stable Coronary Disease. NEJM. April 7, 2005, Volume 352:1425-1435 number 14

42. Jenkins AJ. BMJ 2003 Oct 18;327(7420):933

43. (Almost) Everything You Need To Know About Statin Drugs. Center For Medical Consumers.   www.medicalconsumers.org

44. Cholesterol and mortality: 30 years of follow-up from the Framingham study. JAMA. 1987 Apr 24;257(16):2176-80

45. Cholesterol and the Pharmaceutical Industry's Biggest Secret. www.oqey.com

46. Behar S, Graff E, Reicher-Reiss H, Boyko V, Benderly M, Shotan A, Brunner D. Low total cholesterol is associated with high total mortality in patients with coronary heart disease. The Bezafibrate Infarction Prevention (BIP) Study Group. Eur Heart J. 1997 Jan;18(1):52-9

47. BBC News. Statin fortified drinking water? 01/08/2004

48. Washington Post August 9, 2001

49. Steven E. Nissen, M.D., E. Murat Tuzcu, M.D., Paul Schoenhagen, M.D., Tim Crowe, B.S., William J. Sasiela, Ph.D., John Tsai, M.D., John Orazem, Ph.D., Raymond D. Magorien, M.D., Charles O'Shaughnessy, M.D., Peter Ganz, M.D., for the Reversal of Atherosclerosis with Aggressive Lipid Lowering (REVERSAL) Investigators. The New England Journal of Medicine. Volume 352:29 38. Jan 6, 2005

50. Psychosom Med. 1994 Nov-Dec;56(6):479-84 Demonstration of an association among dietary cholesterol, central serotonergic activity, and social behavior in monkeys. Kaplan JR, Shively CA, Fontenot MB, Morgan TM, Howell SM, Manuck SB, Muldoon MF, Mann JJ.

51. Psychosomatic Medicine 2000;62

52. Golombe al 2004

53. Zhang J, et al. Association of serum cholesterol and history of school suspension among school-aged children and adolescents in the United States. American Journal of Epidemiology, Apr 1, 2005;161(7):691 699

54. Composition of CNS Myelin and Brain. American Society for Neurochemistry. 1999

55. Zhang J, et al. Serum cholesterol concentrations are associated with visuomotor speed in men: findings from the third National Health and Nutrition Examination Survey, 1988-1994. American Journal of Clinical Nutrition, Aug. 2004; 80: 291-298

56. Leardi S, Altilia F, Delmonaco S, et al. 2000. Blood levels of cholesterol and postoperative septic complications. Ann Ital Chir 71 (2):233-237

57. Crook MA, Velauthar U, Moran L, Griffiths W. Hypocholesterolaemia in a hospital population. Ann Clin Biochem. 1999 Sep;36 (Pt 5):613-6

58. Read TE, Harris HW, Grunfeld C, Feingold KR, Kane JP, Rapp JH. The protective effect of serum lipoproteins against bacterial lipopolysaccharide. Eur Heart J. 1993 Dec;14 Suppl K:125-9

59. Horwich TB, Hamilton MA, Maclellan WR, Fonarow GC. Low serum total cholesterol is associated with marked increase in mortality in advanced heart failure. J Card Fail. 2002 Aug;8(4):216-24

60. Ulmer H, et al. Why Eve is not Adam: prospective follow-up in 149 650 women and men of cholesterol and other risk factors related to cardiovascular and all-cause mortality. Journal of Women's Health, Jan-Feb. 2004;13(1):41-53

61. Circulation 1992 86:3:1026-1029

62. Ridker PM, Hennekens CH, Buring JE, Rifai N. C-reactive protein and other markers of inflammation in the prediction of cardiovascular disease in women. NEJM 2000

63. American Heart Association

64. Ross R. Factors influencing atherogenesis. In: Hurst JW, Schlant RC, Rackley CE, Sonnenblick EH, Wenger NK, editors. The heart, arteries and veins. New York: McGraw-Hill, 1990: 877-923

65. Stampfer MJ, Malinow MR, Willet WC, Newcomer LM, Upson B, Ullmann D, et al. A prospective study of plasma homocyst(e)ine and risk of myocardial infarction in US physicians. JAMA 1992;268(7):877-881

66. Miller AL, Kelly GS. Homocysteine Metabolism: Nutritional modulation and impact on health and disease. Alt Med Rev 1997;2(4):234-254

67. Ross R. Factors influencing atherogenesis. In: Hurst JW, Schlant RC, Rackley CE, Sonnenblick EH, Wenger NK, editors. The heart, arteries and veins. New York: McGraw-Hill, 1990: 877-923.

68. Peter Libby, MD; Paul M. Ridker, MD; Attilio Maseri, MD. Inflammation and Atherosclerosis. Circulation 2002;105:1135

69. Sowers JR. Obesity as a cardiovascular risk factor. Am J Med. 2003 Dec 8;115

70. Circulating Mononuclear Cells in the Obese Found to be in Proinflammatory State, Contributing to Diabetes and Heart Disease. University of Buffalo, The State University of New York. 20th September 2004

71. Scott M. Grundy, MD. PhD. Inflammation, Hypertension, and the Metabolic Syndrome. JAMA, December 10, 2003 Vol 290. No 22.

72. Haffner SM, Lehto S, Ronnemaa T et al. Mortality from coronary heart disease in subjects with type 2 diabetes and in nondiabetic subjects with and without prior myocardial infarction. N Engl J Med 1998;339:229-34

Reference

73. Hu FB, Stampfer MJ, Solomon CG et al. The impact of diabetes mellitus on mortality from all causes and coronary heart disease in women. Arch Intern Med 2001;161:1717-23

74. Penninx BWJH, Beekman ATF, Honig A, Deeg DJH, Schoevers RA, van Eijk JTM, van Tilburg W. Depression and cardiac mortality: results from a community-based longitudinal study. Arch Gen Psychiatry 2001;58:221-227

75. Wajed, J. et al. Prevention of cardiovascular disease in systemic lupus erythematosis – proposed guidelines for risk factor management. Rheumatology 2004;43:7-12

76. Kao A et al. Update on vascular disease in systemic lupus erythematosis. Curr Opin Rheumatol 15:519-527

77. Tummala PE, Chen XL, Sundell CL, et al. Angiotensin II induces vascular cell adhesion molecule-1 expression in rat vasculature: a potential link between the renin-angiotensin system and atherosclerosis. Circulation. 1999;100:1223-1229.

78. The New York Times March 8, 2005

79. Cleland JG, et al. The Warfarin/Aspirin Study in Heart failure (WASH):a randomized trial comparing antithrombotic strategies for patients with heart failure. Am Heart J. 2004 Jul;148(1):157-64.

80. Doetsch K, Roheim PS, Thompson JJ. Human lipoprotein (a) quantified by 'capture' ELISA. Ann Clin Lab Sci 1991;21(3):216-218.

81. Bill Statham The Chemical Maze, 2nd edition. Possibility.com 2002

82. Howell WH et al. Plasma lipid and lipoprotein responses to dietary fat and cholesterol: a meta-analysis. Am J Clin Nutr. 75:1084-1092. 1997

83. Malcolm Kendrick, MD. Redflagsweekly.com

84. Prior IA, Davidson F, et. al. "Cholesterol, coconuts, and diet on Polynesian atolls: a natural experiment: the Pukapuka and Tokelau island studies." American Journal of Clinical Nutrition. 1981 Aug;34(8):1552-61

85. Sircar S, Kansra U. J Indian Med Assoc. 1998 Oct;96(10):304-7. Choice of cooking oils--myths and realities

86. Zampelas A, et al. Am J Clin Nutr 2004;80:862-7

87. 22nd Congress of the European Society of Cardiology, August 2000

88. Cortisol's role in weight gain still up for debate. Arizona Central, Mar. 29, 2005

Cholesterol: The Real Tr

References

89. American Journal of Epidemiology February 15, 2001; 153: 353-362
90. MacLatchy et al. The phytoestrogen beta-sitosterol alters the reproductive endocrine status of goldfish. Toxicol Appl Pharmacol. 1995 Oct;134(2):305-12
91. Valerie James, BA. Toxins On Your Toast. The Weston A. Price Foundation
92. Mellanen et al. Wood-derived estrogens: studies in vitro with breast cancer cell lines and in vivo in trout. Toxicol Appl Pharmacol. 1996 Feb;136(2):381-8
93. Rydholm, Pulping Processes. Interscience Publishing, 1965, pp 226 227 & 826-827
94. Richelle M, et al. Both free and esterified plant sterols reduce cholesterol absorption and the bioavailability of beta-carotene and alpha-tocopherol in normocholesterolemic humans. Am J Clin Nutr. 2004 Jul;80(1):171-7
95. www.mercola.com
96. Williams S. Yancy, Jr., MD, MHS; Maren K. Olsen, Ph D; John R. Guyton, MD; Ronna P. Bakst, RD; and Eric C. Westman, MD, MHS. A Low-Carbohydrate, Ketogenic Diet versus a Low-Fat Diet To Treat Obesity and Hyperlipidemia. Ann Intern Med. 2004 May 18;140(10):769-77
97. Pereira MA, et al. Effects of a low-glycaemic load diet on resting energy expenditure and heart disease risk factors during weight loss. JAMA. 2004 Nov 24;292(20):2482-90
98. Leaf A, et al. Cardiovascular effects of n-3 fatty acids. NEJM 1988;318(9),549-57(88).
99. Hu FB, Bronner L, Willett WC, et al. Fish and omega-3 fatty acid intake and risk of coronary heart disease in women. JAMA. 2002;287:1815"1821
100. Nestel P, Shige H, Pomeroy S, et al. The n-3 fatty acids eicosapentanoic acid and docosahexanoic acid increase systemic arterial compliance in humans. Am J Clin Nutr. 2002;76:326"330
101. Harvard School of Public Health
102. BBC News 24-08-2004
103. Grundy S. Influence of stearic acid on cholesterol metabolism relative to other long-chain fatty acids. Am J Clin Nutr 1994;60

(suppl.):986S-90S

104. Inhibition of LDL oxidation by cocoa, Lancet, November 1996; 348(2):1514

105. BMJ 1998;317:1341-1345

106. Wald NJ et al. A strategy to reduce cardiovascular disease by more than 80 percent. BMJ 2003;326:1419-23

107. Oscar H Franco et al. The Polymeal: a more natural, safer and probably tastier (than the Polypill) strategy to reduce cardiovascular disease by more than 75%. BMJ 2004;329:1447-1450 (18 Dec.)

108. Medical Observer Weekly, 13 August 2004

109. Gokce N, Keaney JF Jr, Frei B, et al. Long-term ascorbic acid administration reverses endothelial vasomotor dysfunction in patients with coronary artery disease. Circulation. 1999 Jun 29;99(25):3234-40

110. University of Maryland Medical Center

111. Singh RB, Niaz MA. Serum concentration of lipoprotein (a) decreases on treatment with hydrosoluble coenzyme Q10 in patients with coronary artery disease: discovery of a new role. Int J Cardiol. 1999 Jan;68(1):23-9

112. Circulation, 105;2476:2002

113. Journal of Nutrition, 131;27-32:2001

114. Cao, G., Sofic E., Prior, R.L., Antioxidant capacity of tea and common vegetables. Journal of Agriculture and Food Chemistry, 44, 1996, pages 3426-3431.

115. University of Maryland Medical Center

116. Journal of Nutrition May 2000;130:1124-31

117. University of Maryland Medical Center

118. American Dietetic Association

119. Englisch W, Beckers C, Unkauf M, Ruepp M, Zinserling V. Efficacy of Artichoke dry extract in patients with hyperlipoproteinemia. Arzneimittelforschung. 2000 Mar;50(3):260-5.

120. Brown JE, Rice-Evans CA. Luteolin-rich artichoke extract protects low density lipoprotein from oxidation in vitro. Free Radic Res. 1998 Sep;29(3):247-55

121. F.M. Fennessy, MB, BCh, PhD; D.S. Moneley, MB, AFRCSI; J.H. Wang, MB, BCli, PhD; C.J. Kelly, MB, MCh; D.J. Bouchier Hayes, MB, MCh, FRCS. Taurine and vitamin C modify monocyte

and endothelial dysfunction in young smokers. Circulation, Jan 2003; 107: 410 - 415.

122. Wittstein, I.S. and H.C. Champion. 2005. Neurohumoral features of myocardial stunning due to sudden emotional stress. New England Journal of Medicine 352(Feb. 10):539-548

23. Yale-New Haven Hospital. Sleep imbalance linked to heart disease

24. The Australian, 08 March 2005

25. True love keeps heart beating. The Weekend Australian 21 March 05

26. Mildred S. Seeling, MD. Consequences of magnesium deficiency on the enhancement of stress reactions; preventive and therapeutic implications (a review). Journal of the American College of Nutrition, Vol. 13, No. 5, 429-446 (1994).

27. Walker, R. The Cell Factor. Pan Macmillan, Sydney. 2003

28. Journal of Sports Medicine and Physical Fitness December 2001;41:539-545

29. Annual Meeting of the Society of Psychophysiological Research in Montreal, Canada. Oct 18, 2001

30. IM Lee, RS Paffenbarger. Associations of light, moderate, and vigorous intensity physical activity with longevity - The Harvard Alumni Health Study. American Journal of Epidemiology, 2000, Vol 151, Iss 3, pp 293-299

1. Reuters November 30, 2004

2. Kime, Zane R. Sunlight Could Save Your Life. World Health Publications, 1980

3. Knutsson, A., et al., 'Increased Risk of Ischaemic Heart Disease in Shift Workers', Lancet: 11; 89-92, 1986.

4. Meeting of the American Heart Association's Council for High Blood Pressure Research October 2000

5. Tomi-Pekka Tuomainen, research fellow,a Riitta Salonen, senior clinical research fellow,a Kristiina Nyyssönen, clinical biochemist,a Jukka T Salonen, academy professor of Academy of Finland. Cohort study of relation between donating blood and risk of myocardial infarction in 2682 men in Eastern Finland. BMJ 1997;314:793 (15 March).

Index

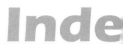

Index

chocolate 28, 130-131, 156, 165

chylomicron 19, 48

cigarettes 41, 90, 155

Co enzyme Q10 56, 134-135

coconut 16, 28, 43, 155, 164
    benefits of 108-109

coffee 83, 102, 109-110

cognitive function 75
    effect of statins on 62

coronary 49-51, 89, 98-99, 148, 167

C-reactive protein 55, 70, 80-81, 87, 91-93, 121, 129, 134, 142
    blood test for 100

creatine kinase 58, 73, 167

dandelion root 140-141

depression 18, 36, 39, 45, 91, 145, 150
    side effect of cholesterol lowering drugs 62-63
    symptom of low cholesterol 75

diabetes 23, 37, 81, 150
    as a cause of excessive inflammation 89-90
    blood test for 100

eggs 16-17, 22, 82, 88, 107-108, 119, 138, 161, 164

exercise 50, 58, 148-151, 156
    lack of exercise as a cause of high cholesterol 40-41

fibrate 58, 61, 63, 73, 130

fiber 160, 163, 166
    lack of fiber as a cause of high cholesterol 34
    to reduce cholesterol 121-122

fish oil 44, 93, 123-125

flaxseed oil 44, 95, 123-125, 155, 164

folic acid 82-83, 91, 101, 130, 132, 138

frying 28, 30, 33, 45, 88, 108

garlic 95, 133, 137, 143, 159, 162, 165

ginger 137, 158, 165

globe artichoke 141

green tea 136, 156, 158, 165

HDL 20, 35, 40-41, 72-73, 90, 119, 124, 150
    blood test for 97-99
    effects of trans fats on 32, 127, 155

heart attack 21, 37-38, 41, 51-52, 80-81, 83, 145-147, 152, 169

Heart Association
    recommendations for "at risk" individuals 98-100

high blood pressure 40, 72, 84, 99, 150
    as a cause of excessive inflammation 93
    diagnosis of Syndrome X 35
    test for 101-102

HMG-Co A reductase 15, 37, 55-56

homocysteine 91, 110, 132, 138, 168-169
    blood test for 101

Index

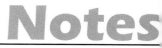

Notes

Notes

Note

Notes

Other Books by Sandra Cabot MD

The Liver Cleansing Diet

Dr Cabot's best selling book which opened the eyes of
millions around the world to the importance of the liver
in maintaining good health. An eight week diet; vital
principles for improving liver function and many liver
friendly recipes to incorporate into your life are provided.

Can't Lose Weight?
Unlock the Secrets that keep you Fat

A revolutionary book that reveals ALL the hidden medical
reasons why people cannot lose weight. The book
provides a 12 week weight loss plan specifically designed
to treat Syndrome X, also called insulin resistance, or
metabolic syndrome.

Raw Juices Can Save Your Life

Dr Cabot says "I have seen juicing work miracles in some o
my patients who were stuck on the merry-go-round of dru
therapy". This book is an A to Z guide of juicing recipes fo
many different health conditions.

The Body Shaping Diet

Learn to identify which body type you have and how this
affects your weight and your hormones. Each body type
has unique patterns of weight gain, hormone levels and
food cravings. A weight loss eating plan is provided for
each of the four body types.

The Healthy Liver and Bowel Book

Specific, life saving strategies are outlined for a number of bowel and liver diseases, including hepatitis, gallstones, cirrhosis, irritable bowel syndrome, diverticulitis and many more. Over 100 new liver cleansing recipes are included.

Hormone Replacement: The Real Truth

This book gives you up to date information on the latest options in hormone replacement therapy. From dietary changes and herbal remedies to bio-identical hormone creams; all of your options are explored. Learn how to restore your libido, beat hot flashes and get a better night's sleep.

Boost Your Energy

Find out how to recharge the energy factories within your cells and fine tune the body and mind with powerful anti-aging hormones and immune boosting nutrients. A 14 day energy diet is provided . Learn how to overcome energy draining conditions such as chronic fatigue syndrome and fibromyalgia and recharge your adrenal glands.